Local Anaesthesia in Dentistry

Senior commissioning editor: Mary Seager
Editorial assistant: Caroline Savage
Production controller: Anthony Read
Desk editor: Angela Davies
Cover designer: Fred Rose

Local Anaesthesia in Dentistry

Paul D. Robinson PhD BDS MBBS FDS
Senior Lecturer/Consultant
Division of Oral and Maxillofacial Surgery
Guy's King's and St Thomas' Dental Institute
King's College
London, UK

Thomas R. Pitt Ford PhD BDS FDS
Professor of Endontology
Division of Conservative Dentistry
Guy's King's and St Thomas' Dental Institute
King's College
London, UK

and

Fraser McDonald PhD MSc BDS FDS MOrth
Professor of Oral Biology/Honorary Consultant
Division of Orthodontics and Paediatric Dentistry
Guy's King's and St Thomas' Dental Institute
King's College
London, UK

wright

OXFORD   AUCKLAND   BOSTON   JOHANNESBURG   MELBOURNE   NEW DELHI

Wright
An imprint of Butterworth-Heinemann
Linacre House, Jordan Hill, Oxford OX2 8DP
225 Wildwood Avenue, Woburn, MA 01801-2041
A division of Reed Educational and Professional Publishing Ltd

Ɋ A member of the Reed Elsevier plc group

First published 2000
Reprinted 2001

British Library Cataloguing in Publication Data
Robinson, Paul D.
    Local anaesthesia in dentistry
    1. Anesthesia in dentistry   2. Local anethesia
    I. Title   II. Pitt Ford, T. R.   III. McDonald, F. (Fraser)
    617.9′676

Library of Congress Cataloguing in Publication Data
A catalogue record for this book is available from the Library of Congress

ISBN 0 7236 1063 0

For information on all Butterworth-Heinemann publications
please visit our website at www.bh.com

Typeset by E & M Graphics, Midsomer Norton, Bath
Printed and bound by MPG Books Ltd, Bodmin, Cornwall

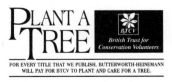

FOR EVERY TITLE THAT WE PUBLISH, BUTTERWORTH-HEINEMANN
WILL PAY FOR BTCV TO PLANT AND CARE FOR A TREE.

Contents

Preface

Local anaesthesia is probably one of the most undervalued aspects of modern clinical practice, yet is the cornerstone to sound patient management. The intention of this book, which was inspired by the original book by Howe and Whitehead, was to provide a small affordable textbook capable of fitting into the pocket of a clinical tunic or coat. It is aimed intentionally for the clinical student embarking upon their first clinical experiences; the second year undergraduate. It is also hoped, however, that the first year 'pre-clinical' students will see an immediate value of anatomy and physiology. There are 11 small chapters beginning with the direct application of clinical science in the first two chapters; how a nerve works and how the anaesthetic solution obstructs this. Obviously equipment is essential, and we have tried to provide the latest syringes currently available. We then tried to detail each aspect of this technique and have tried to emphasize a sound clinical approach that will deal with the vast majority of clinical situations. We finished with a chapter on the actual 'problem-based' philosophy showing the typical litigation resulting from the use of local anaesthesia. By the limitations of size and cost we were not able to cover every aspect and we hope to have directed the student to further larger textbooks and, where appropriate, evidence-based articles at the end of each chapter.

Paul D. Robinson
Thomas R. Pitt Ford
Fraser McDonald

Chapter 1

Physiology of nerve conduction

Local anaesthesia has developed through the last 100 years so that achievement of effective anaesthesia is simple and predictable. As a consequence complex and highly technical procedures in dentistry have become possible. There is no doubt that the general public perceives a good dentist as a practitioner causing little or no discomfort. In turn, general dental practitioners identify a good anaesthetic as one that allows them to focus solely on the operative procedure without distractions from pain-induced patient movements. The everyday practice of dentistry is therefore based upon a sound local anaesthetic technique.

Pain is abolished by interrupting the pathways that carry the information of the stimulus from the periphery of the body to the central nervous system, or by removing the stimulus. The pain of dental treatment is associated, on the majority of occasions, with the stimulus of instrumentation, which by definition cannot be stopped. The obstruction of the sensory pathways that provoke a pain response can be achieved by the application of an anaesthetic solution to the sensory nerves supplying the area of stimulation. In this way a localised area of the body is anaesthetised but the patient remains conscious, i.e. local anaesthesia.

This chapter considers the general physiology of nerve conduction. The complexities of pain conduction will be considered only at the local level; conduction within higher centres, and theories of pain perception, are beyond the scope of this book. Later chapters describe the basic delivery of local anaesthesia. Specific words have been defined in the glossary at the end of the book to assist the student in understanding the terminology.

Local nerve conduction

Throughout the body there is a vast network involved with the transmission of information: the nervous system. This carries information rapidly throughout the body at speeds well beyond those of other messenger systems. Not only does the system carry information

Table 1.1   The basic characteristics and classification of fibre diameters of nerves

Fibre type	Function	Fibre diameter (μm)
A α	Proprioception, somatic motor	12–20
β	Touch, pressure	5–12
γ	Motor to muscle spindles	3–6
δ	Pain, cold, touch	2–5
B	Preganglionic autonomic	< 3
C	Pain, temperature, mechanosensitive	0.4–1.2
Sympathetic	Postganglionic sympathetic	0.3–1.3

from the periphery of the body to the central nervous system (sensory and proprioceptive information) but it also responds to that information (motor response).

Nervous tissue, motor and sensory, has many forms depending on its structure and dimensions (Table 1.1), which in turn modify certain aspects of function.

The overall form of a nerve is illustrated in Figure 1.1. The central core, or nerve fibre, acts like the metal found within household wire, conducting electrical activity. The myelin sheath is essentially an insulator, similar to the plastic surrounding the wire, but with gaps found within this covering: the nodes of Ranvier. These nodes allow rapid passage of the excitatory impulse along the nerve, effectively jumping from one node to the next (saltatory conduction). This passage of information as an impulse is known as 'propagation of an action potential', and the physiology of the nervous tissue producing this active or action potential is the basis of understanding how local anaesthetics work. Nerve cells contact each other at junctions known as synapses, which serve to coordinate nervous activity and ensure unidirectional flow of electrical activity.

The basis of the action potential is derived from the balance of ions that produce the resting membrane potential. In non-activated nervous tissue, there is a distribution of ions across the membrane produced by a protein which distributes sodium ions (Na^+) outside the cell and potassium ions (K^+) inside the cell. The normal distribution of these ions across a semi-permeable membrane would distribute equal amounts of Na^+ and K^+ either side. However, under the influence of adenosine triphosphate (ATP), ion exchange takes place; 3 Na^+ are removed for every 2 K^+ imported into the cell. The molecule responsible for this active exchange is referred to as a Na^+-K^+ *ATPase*. Each movement of ions is associated with hydrolysis of one molecule of ATP.

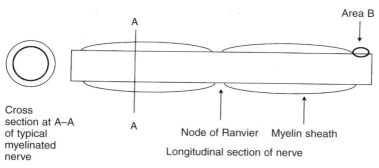

Figure 1.1.   A diagrammatic representation of a typical myelinated nerve. At the nodes of Ranvier (Area B) ion channels and electrogenic pumps are found crossing the membrane. A diagram of these is shown in Figure 1. 2A.

The mechanism, often referred to as an electrogenic pump, continues throughout the life of the cell.

The typical resulting distribution of ions produces a membrane potential that is equivalent to –70 mV (Table 1.2) and can be calculated by an equation which relates the concentration of *multiple* ions either side of a membrane with the electrical potential across that membrane (Goldmann equation). This is often considered with a further equation, which relates the membrane potential to the concentration of a *single* ion either side of a cell membrane (Nernst equation). The concentration of chloride ions (Cl^-) is also often quoted, as they are the main electronegative ions, contributing to the electrical neutrality of the cell and to volume regulation through osmosis.

Diameter of nerves

In addition to ionic characteristics, nerves also have varying diameters. The fibre diameters of nerves are a major factor in determining the

Table 1.2   The distribution of ions responsible for the resting membrane potential of a nerve

Ion	Concentration Mmol / l of H_2O		Equilibrium potential (mV)
	Inside	Outside	
Na+	15	150	+60
K+	150	4	–90
Cl⁻	9	125	–70

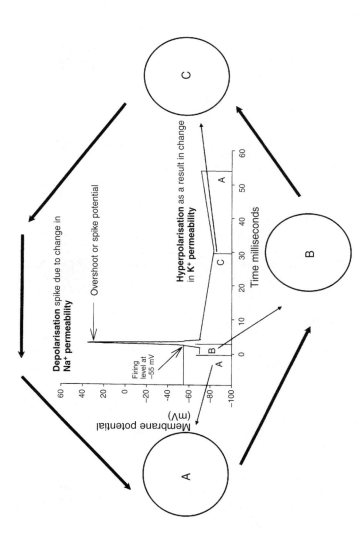

Figure 1.2. The changes in the membrane potential of a myelinated nerve. The insets demonstrate the changes found during the passage of an action potential: A represents the resting membrane potential with only the Na^+-K^+ ATPase pump modifying ionic balance; B represents the initial changes with a major change in Na^+ permeability; C represents the slower change in K^+ permeability.

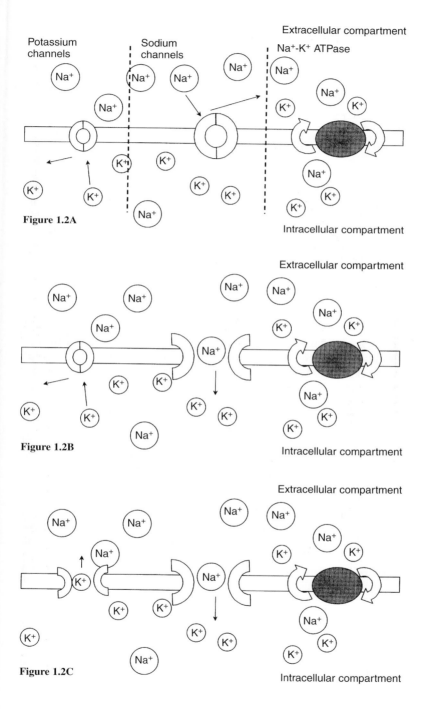

Figure 1.2A

Figure 1.2B

Figure 1.2C

speed of conduction. They are classified as A, B or C; A having the largest diameter (Table 1.1).

Ion channels

These structures are proteins which span the cell membrane, allowing the passage of discrete molecules/ions across the lipid bilayer. They number several million per mm^2 of membrane. Normally the lipid bilayer allows only fat-soluble molecules through by diffusion, and blocks polar water-soluble molecules and ions. The ion channels are the mechanism by which these water-soluble molecules/ions can pass into or out of the cells. The channels are often specific for different types of ions (typically Na^+, K^+, Cl^- and Ca^{2+}). They exist in open or closed conditions, being opened (gated) by membrane potential (voltage gated) or by the actions of biochemical substances/hormones (often collectively referred to as agonists) on receptors.

Passage of an action potential

Following stimulation there is a change in ion distribution, which in turn alters the membrane potential. The response of the nerve depends on the extent of change in this potential. If the ionic distribution varies minimally then the Na^+-K^+ ATPase protein will restore the change in potential to the resting value, and no action potential will be produced. If, however, the change in potential reaches a critical figure (-55 mV), there is a major change in the permeability of the plasma membrane, and proteins within the membrane become distorted and allow passage of Na^+ ions only. From Table 1.2 it can be seen that the concentration of Na^+ ions is highest outside the cell; so these will rush into the cell, causing a rapid change (in 1–2 milliseconds) in potential to approximately +30 mV. Much slower (9–10 milliseconds) than this is a change in K^+ permeability. The ion channels span the plasma membrane, and their specific structures are now being identified. It is these proteins which appear to be blocked by local anaesthetic solutions. The typical characteristics are seen in Figure 1.2, which shows the changes in membrane potential over time in a nerve (stimulated by an external electrical source in this case).

The changes in membrane potential

The action potential demonstrated in Figure 1.2 can be described in three basic areas: at rest (A); change in Na^+ permeability (B); and change in K^+ permeability (C). For clarity the insets demonstrate specific features.

A The resting membrane potential of −70 m is maintained by the balance of Na^+, K^+ and Cl^- ions, and can be calculated using the Goldmann equation.

B The first change in ion balance is as a consequence of the membrane potential reaching 55 mV (the firing level or threshold). At this level the Na^+ from outside the cell passes into the cell through voltage-gated sodium channels along the ion's concentration gradient. This takes the membrane potential to +30 mV, approaching the equilibrium potential of Na^+, i.e. +60 mV (Table 1.2). The +60 mV is not reached because:
  1. The influx of Na^+ is short-lived (1–2 ms), the channel closing soon after activation.
  2. The electrical gradient for Na^+ is reversed, thus preventing further overshoot.
  3. The slower voltage-gated K^+ channels open.

C The 'after-hyperpolarization' occurs solely due to the changes in K^+ permeability. The voltage-gated K+ channels act more slowly and for a more prolonged period, leading to a loss of positive charge out of the cell.

Molecular basis of pain

The events leading to the sensation of pain at the cellular level often involve tissue damage, whether infective or traumatic (either physical, thermal or chemical). These insults to the tissues will provoke localised inflammation, which produces the cardinal signs of redness, heat, swelling, pain and immobility.

A number of molecules and ions have been identified in the inflammatory process:

1. Cytokines (interleukins and growth factors). Many cell types, including lymphocytes, osteoblasts and macrophages produce these molecules. Their action in producing inflammation and (potentially) pain may be either direct, or indirect by stimulating the production of prostaglandins.
2. Histamine. This is a potent vasoactive amine released from mast cells, in high concentrations producing either pruritus (mildly irritating stimulation often referred to as itch) or pain. Another substance provoking pain and produced by mast cells is 5-hydroxy-tryptamine (serotonin).

3. Ionic imbalances (potassium and hydrogen). Both these ions can cause pain when present in high concentrations. In the case of K^+ in particular, this can reflect lysis of cells as it is a major intracellular ion. In addition high concentrations of K^+ can cause hyperexcitability of nerves, effectively lowering the firing threshold.
4. Substance P. This substance, often found as a neurotransmitter, is a known stimulator of vasodilatation and lysosymal activation.
5. Prostaglandins and related metabolites. Prostaglandin E is most associated with pain and inflammation. Leukotrienes are often discussed in association with prostaglandins, especially leukotriene B_4, which can also stimulate pain. Both these substances are metabolites of arachidonic acid.

There are two basic theories of pain generation. In the first it is believed that the normal senses are stimulated to such a degree that pain is a consequence. The simplest example is that of the continuing application of heat. The initial applications, though sensed, will not cause pain as there is no tissue damage. As the temperature increases so pain occurs, as proteins are released by tissue damage. The second theory is centred on a specific 'pain' system throughout the organism, which identifies as pain all stimuli evoking tissue damage; this latter theory, however, is less well supported by research.

Blockade of the nervous pathways is the basis of local anaesthetic action. This is described in Chapter 2.

Suggested further reading

Ganong, W. F. (1997). *Review of Medical Physiology*, 18th edition. Appleton and Lange, Connecticut, USA.
Meechan, J. G., Robb, N. D., Seymour, R. A. (1998). *Pain and Anxiety Control for the Conscious Dental Patient*. Oxford University Press.

Chapter 2

Pharmacological basis of local anaesthesia

The general constituents of a cartridge of anaesthetic solution are:

1. local anaesthetic agent
2. vasoconstrictor
3. reducing agent
4. preservative
5. fungicide
6. carrier solution.

In combination these produce a solution which is effective, non-toxic and biocompatible, being isotonic with the tissues and of comparable pH. In addition the solution and its constituents need to be sterile and to have a long shelf life. The constituents will be considered in turn.

Local anaesthetic agent

Molecular basis of local anaesthesia

It appears that all local anaesthetic agents work by obstructing the change in Na^+ permeability, essential for the initial phases of the action potential. In this manner the wave of depolarisation which passes along the nerve is either prevented from developing, or if already initiated along the nerve fibre, prevented from propagating further. Local anaesthetics may have their effect on the channels both internally and externally to the nerve membrane. Some however seem to affect only the internal aspect, as their hydrophobic properties allow them to pass through the myelin sheath and across the cell membrane to interfere with Na^+ permeability from within the axon. In this way the voltage-gated Na^+ channels are inactivated.

The movement of Na^+ ions may also be modified in a non-specific manner. The high lipid solubility of the agents may modify the membrane structure preventing the normal function of the nerves.

Pharmacological characteristics

The local anaesthetic agents are classified according to their basic chemical structure (Table 2.1) and consist of a 'water-repellent' (hydrophobic) part of a molecule, an intermediate linking chain, and a 'water-attractant' (hydrophilic) part of a molecule. The combination of parts of the molecules that repel or attract water are essential for the compounds to act correctly; not only by dissolving correctly, but also by diffusing through the tissues of the body. The intermediate chain separating the hydrophilic and hydrophobic ends is either an amide or an ester-based link. The earlier agents, procaine and cocaine, were ester-based; these drugs are no longer in widespread use as dental local anaesthetics because of unwanted side effects (toxicity and allergy: see Chapter 10). Different local anaesthetic drugs have varying proportions of hydrophilic and hydrophobic components. These differences modify the characteristics and/or properties of the anaesthetic agents in the following areas:

1. intrinsic anaesthetic potency
2. duration of action
3. effects on other tissues (toxicity)
4. rate of degradation, both locally and systemically.

Intrinsic anaesthetic potency

The minimum concentration of a local anaesthetic agent required to reduce the nerve potential by half its amplitude within 5 minutes is a measure of the intrinsic potency. It is a measure of the pharmacological action of the agent.

Onset of anaesthesia

The onset of anaesthesia is dependent on the speed at which the agent passes through the tissues and acts on the target nerves. The closer the solution is placed to the nerve to be anaesthetised, the more rapid is the onset of anaesthesia. The diameter of the nerve fibre also determines the rate of diffusion into the site of action within the nerve bundle (sheath). The smaller nerves, which tend to be mainly sensory, are affected more rapidly than the larger nerves.

Duration of action

After arrival of the anaesthetic at the ion channels, the active agent will then diffuse away from the area. Duration of anaesthesia is dependent on the rate of diffusion along a concentration gradient away from the

Table 2.1   Formulation of local anaesthetic agents

Main anaesthetic agent	Commercial name and manufacturer	Ampoule size		Vasoconstrictor	Concentration
Lignocaine 2% (Lidocaine – USA)	Xylocaine: Astra	2.2 ml	(1.8 ml USA)	Adrenaline	1:80,000
	Lignostab: Atra	2.2 ml		None	(In USA 1:100.000 or 1:50,000)
	Lignospan: Septodont	2.2 ml			
Articaine 4%	Septonest: Septodont	1.7 ml		Adrenaline	1:100,000; 1:200,000
Prilocaine 4%	Citanest: Astra	2.2 ml		None	
Prilocaine 3%	Citanest: Astra	2.2 ml		Felypressin	0.03 IU/ml
Mepivacaine 3%	Scandonest: Septodont	2.2 ml		None	
Mepivicaine 2%	Scandonest: Septodont	2.2 ml		Adrenaline	1:200,000
Bupivacaine 0.25%	Marcain: Astra	10 ml		None	
Bupivacaine 0.25%	Marcain: Astra	10 ml		Adrenaline	1:200,000
Cream:					
Lignocaine 2.5% and prilocaine 2.5%	Emla: Astra	30 g tube			

nerve and into the tissue space, and then into the blood vessels. It is also dependent on the concentration of solution around the nerves and the number of blood vessels (arterioles, capillaries and venules). In highly vascular sites, such as the posterior maxilla, anaesthesia is of shorter duration. Inflammation of tissue may also reduce duration, as there is local vasodilatation due to the presence of vasoactive substances.

The most commonly used local anaesthetic agents are lignocaine and prilocaine. There are many other anaesthetic agents, and use of articaine and bupivicaine appears to be increasing. Articaine has a duration of approximately 60 minutes (and other properties support its use); the duration of bupivacaine is considerably longer at 8–10 hours, thus providing postoperative analgesia.

Effects on other tissues (toxicity)

Toxic effects are considered in Chapter 10.

Degradation

The local anaesthetic agent is broken down by dealkylation and hydrolysis. The breakdown products are then conjugated with glucuronic acid. The constituents of the solutions can be degraded locally within the tissues to a limited extent. The majority of the drug is degraded in the liver and the conjugated compounds are excreted.

Variations of this process include the modification of prilocaine in the lungs and kidneys, and the breakdown of articaine by plasma esterases to the metabolite articaine acid, which in turn is conjugated to glucuronic acid.

Excretion

Excretion occurs mainly through removal of conjugated metabolites from the blood by the kidneys. These are discharged into the urine along with a small amount of unchanged agent (< 2%). The anaesthetic agents are generally cleared from the body in 12–24 hours.

Vasoconstrictor

This is included to delay removal of the agent from the tissues through diffusion into local blood vessels. This produces advantages including:

- The duration of anaesthesia is longer with a vasoconstrictor.
- Bleeding is reduced in surgical procedures.
- Systemic toxic effects may be reduced.

Various concentrations of vasoconstrictor and local anaesthetic are currently available (Table 2.1).

The commonest vasoconstrictors used are:

Adrenaline (epinephrine)
Adrenaline acts on α adrenergic receptors found on smooth muscle cells of arterioles promoting contraction of the muscle cell, constriction of the arteriole and a reduction in supply to the capillary bed. There are also effects on β adrenergic receptors mainly in other tissues including striated and cardiac muscle.

Felypressin (Octapressin)
This is a synthetic derivative of oxytocin, and may also cause uterine smooth muscle contraction, but not at the concentration used in local anaesthesia.

Reducing agent

Sodium metabisulphite is included to prevent the oxidation of the vasoconstrictor and acts by competing with adrenaline for the available oxygen dissolved in the solution.

Preservative

The shelf life of local anaesthetics without preservative is approximately 18 months to 2 years. A preservative prolongs the shelf life of the solution, but as most preservatives can provoke allergic reactions these compounds are in fact seldom used. Typical examples include methylparaben solutions and caprylhydrocuprienotoxin.

Fungicide

Thymol is occasionally used in some solutions as a fungicide.

Carrier solution

This is a modified form of Ringer's lactate solution, adjusted for a biocompatible pH.

Further reading

Malamed, S. F. (1990). *Handbook of Local Anaesthesia*. Mosby, St Louis, Los Angeles.

Evers, H., Haegerstam, G. (1990). *Introduction to Dental Local Anaesthesia*. Mediglobe, Fribourg, Switzerland.

Chapter 3

Instruments

Cartridges

Local anaesthetic solution for dentistry is supplied in special cartridges that fit into purpose-made syringes (Figure 3.1), to which specific needles are fitted.

The cartridges have traditionally been made from glass, but have more recently been made from polypropylene (Figure 3.2a, b). They contain 1.8–2.2 ml, the volume of which depends on the solution, manufacturer and market; 1.8 ml is usually sufficient for most dental procedures.

At one end is a thin rubber diaphragm, through which the needle penetrates; at the other is a rubber bung, which is displaced by the

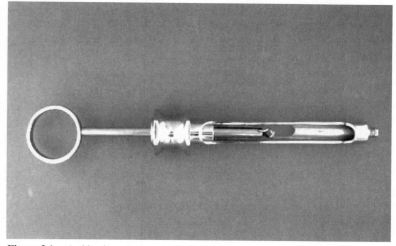

Figure 3.1. A side view of an aspirating syringe showing the handle for placement of the thumb and the harpoon for insertion into the cartridge bung. For many reasons, this type of syringe has been superseded by the type in Figure 3.3.

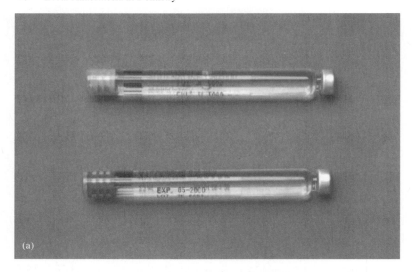

(a)

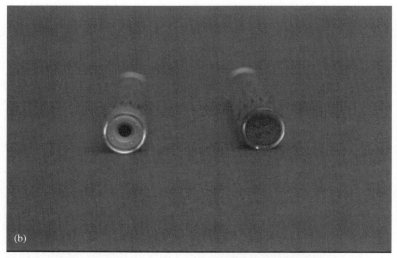

(b)

Figure 3.2.   (a) Two cartridges, one glass and one propylene, containing anaesthetic solution. (b) The cartridges seen from the end of the cartridge into which the plunger fits; on the left is the diaphragm with a specifically designed insert for use by the syringe in Figure 3.3.

plunger of the syringe. For many years the bung was simply pushed by the blunt-ended plunger. The bung was later designed to be harpooned by a barbed tip on the plunger, in order to allow aspiration of fluid (i.e. blood from inadvertent vessel penetration) from the tissues prior to injection. Most recently the bung has had a thin diaphragm in the centre, which can be displaced by a specially shaped plunger; this allows aspiration without the ability to draw up any significant volume into the cartridge (Figure 3.3).

The diaphragm and bung are made from rubber; natural latex is not used, so there should be no risk of allergy in a latex-sensitive patient.

Needles

The needles are supplied in two lengths, 20 mm or 35 mm; the short ones are intended for infiltration procedures while the long ones are for deeper penetration of the tissues in regional block anaesthesia. Needles may come as 27 or 30 gauge, are made from stainless steel, and have a sharp bevelled tip. For many years now dental local anaesthetic needles have been supplied as disposable for single use, and are supplied presterilized. The needles are produced in a two-part sheath (Figure

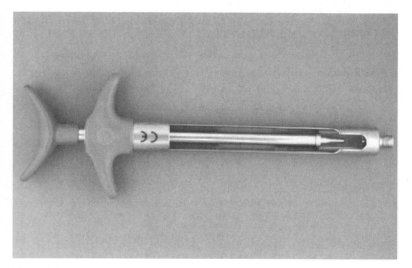

Figure 3.3.   A syringe which will allow pressure to be applied to the cartridge bung, allowing aspiration when the pressure is released. See text for details.

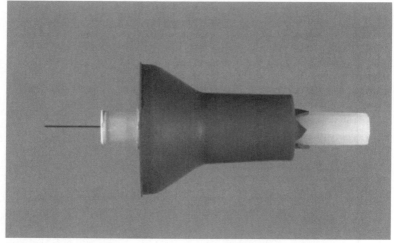

Figure 3.4.   A syringe partially sheathed in a needle guard. The needle guards are used to prevent 'needle stick' injury.

3.4), which is broken by twisting; the plastic hub is then screwed onto the syringe until it is tight.

Syringe

A syringe in simple terms consists of a barrel and a plunger; it is normally made from metal. A needle is fitted to one end of the barrel, and a cartridge is then placed into the barrel, which has one or two windows so that the inside of the cartridge can be observed during use. The plunger fits against the back of the bung in the cartridge. When pressure is applied to the plunger, the bung is moved along the cartridge and solution comes out of the needle. At one time the plunger had a harpoon on its end to engage the rubber bung (Figure 3.1), allowing aspiration to occur. Misuse of this to draw up solutions other than local anaesthetics has resulted in the development of the alternative safe aspiration system described above.

Method of use

The surface anaesthetic should be applied to the appropriate mucosa and allowed to act for approximately 2 minutes before injection. When an injection is to be given, the remaining sheath is removed from the needle and light pressure is placed on the plunger to fill the needle with solution. The needle can then be introduced into the tissues; it is good practice never to insert the needle completely to its hub, as it is weakest at this point. Before the solution is deposited, the plunger should be lightly depressed then released; this will allow aspiration of fluid from the tissues. If blood is aspirated, the needle should be moved and aspiration repeated before injection in order to avoid intravascular placement of the local anaesthetic solution. Should it be necessary to give a further injection to the same patient at that appointment, the needle may be reused, as can the cartridge of anaesthetic solution. After completion of an injection the needle should be resheathed, taking care not to cause a needle-stick injury to the operator or an assistant (see Figure 3.4). At the conclusion of the treatment, the needle and cartridge must be disposed of safely in a suitable 'sharps container' so that there is no re-use on another patient, thus eliminating any risk of cross-infection.

Particular syringes are available for certain purposes, for example an intraligamentary injection (Figure 3.5). They are used rarely compared with the standard syringe. Their main difference is that they have a ratchet device that allows the plunger to move the bung along the cartridge when considerable pressure is needed, because of tissue pressure resistance.

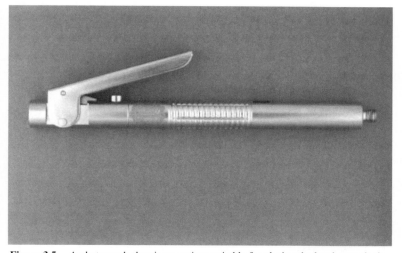

Figure 3.5. A photograph showing a syringe suitable for placing the local anaesthetic solution within the periodontal ligament space: an intraligamental injection. Note that the cartridge is effectively encased to prevent damage from fracture of the glass barrel due to the high injection pressure.

Sterilization

Local anaesthetic needles are supplied presterilized in a two-part sheath. If the seal on the sheath is damaged the needle should not be used. Re-usable needles have not been used for many years.

Cartridges of local anaesthetic contain the solution presterilized and are supplied in blister packs; it is important that the diaphragm end of the cartridge is not contaminated before use.

The syringe must be autoclaved before use so that infection is not transmitted from one patient to another. There is no place for disinfectants in the sterilization of local anaesthetic instruments.

Chapter 4

Techniques for delivery of local anaesthesia

Infiltration anaesthesia and regional block anaesthesia

There are two basic strategies for nerve blockade using local anaesthesia: the infiltration technique and the regional block technique. The patterns of anaesthesia that result are different, and thus the indications for using each method are different, according to the nature of the planned procedure and its site in the mouth. Other factors such as the age of the patient and their level of co-operation may also have a bearing on the technique chosen.

Infiltration technique

Sensory nerves divide into smaller branches that subdivide further before reaching sensory receptors in the tissues. Placement of local anaesthetic solution close to the tissues to be anaesthetised (in this case the teeth and periodontal tissues) allows diffusion of the solution around the fine branches of sensory nerves that supply these areas. Thus the resulting zone of anaesthesia is limited to those structures which are innervated by the network of fine nerve branches and their receptors that are infiltrated by the local anaesthetic at the site of injection (Figure 4.1).

The simplest example of this principle is anaesthetising the pulps of maxillary teeth. Local anaesthetic solution placed in the soft tissues of the vestibule, buccal to the upper teeth readily diffuses through the thin buccal cortex of the maxilla to reach the apices of the teeth and their radicular nerves (Figure 4.2).

Infiltration anaesthesia has a high rate of success (see also Chapter 9) provided that there are no physical barriers to diffusion of the local anaesthetic solution into the tissues to be anaesthetised. A good example of this problem is the thick cortical bone of the posterior mandible in adults, which does not normally permit penetration of the local anaesthetic solution.

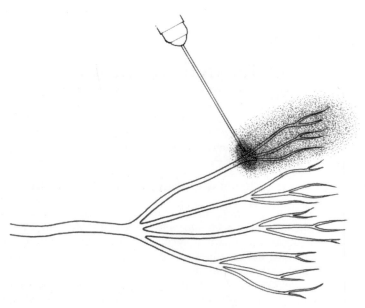

Figure 4.1. Diagrammatic representation of the principle of infiltration anaesthesia showing the anaesthetised area confined to the zone of injection. The stippled area represents the area of anaesthesia.

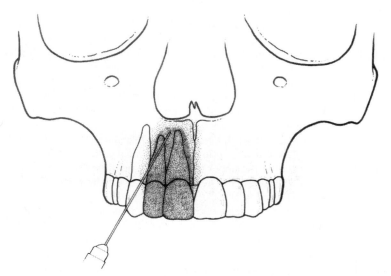

Figure 4.2. Diagram showing an infiltration injection to anaesthetise the right maxillary incisors.

Regional block technique

Placement of local anaesthetic solution around the main trunk of a sensory nerve or one of its major branches blocks all sensory input from the whole region of tissues supplied by that nerve. Regional block anaesthesia therefore tends to affect a wider area than the infiltration technique (Figure 4.3). This has the advantage that more teeth (or other tissues) can be anaesthetised with a single injection, but with the disadvantage that more unwanted soft tissue anaesthesia, e.g. of the lips or tongue, may result.

The site of injection for regional block anaesthesia is usually remote from the teeth to be anaesthetized. In this way, any localised infection in the tissues surrounding the tooth can be avoided by the local anaesthetic needle and the risk of the injection spreading the infection is minimised. Accurate placement of the local anaesthetic solution at the correct anatomical site is essential for the nerve block to be successful. Injections given in the wrong place are a common cause for the failure of regional block anaesthesia.

Some areas of the mouth can only be anaesthetised adequately by regional blocks, e.g. the mandibular permanent molar teeth (Figure 4.4a, b). Blockade of the inferior alveolar nerve can be achieved at the mandibular foramen on the medial aspect of the ramus before the

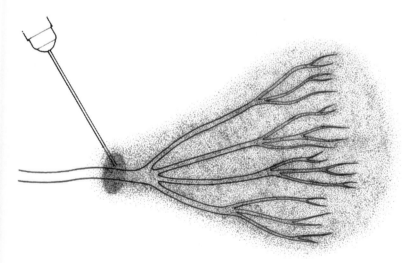

Figure 4.3. Diagrammatic representation of the principle of regional block anaesthesia showing the anaesthetised area involving all of the nerve distribution distal to the point of injection.

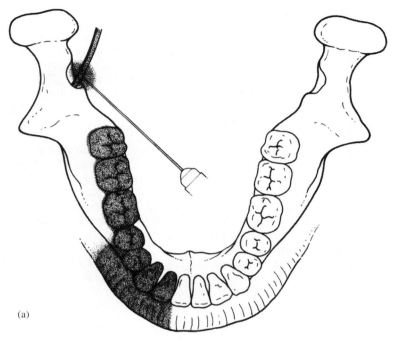

(a)

Figure 4.4.   Regional block anaesthesia involving the body of the mandible and the teeth and lower lip. (a) The site of placement of the anaesthetic is seen close to the mandibular foramen on the medial aspect of the mandibular body. The extent of anaesthesia is shown by the stippling. Note that the mucosa on the lingual aspect of the teeth is not included but the distribution of the mental nerve is. (b) The side view of the area of hard tissue anaesthesia included in the regional block.

nerve enters its canal in the dense bone of the mandibular body, which precludes the use of infiltration techniques at this site.

Preparation for the injection

The patient

Most patients are somewhat fearful of injections; a minority are terrified at the thought of needles. Almost universally the expectation is worse than the reality. Reassurance given to patients and trust gained will often allay their fears. The approach to this begins as the patient enters the surgery with a welcome greeting to an environment that should reflect friendliness and calm, as well as professional competence. A

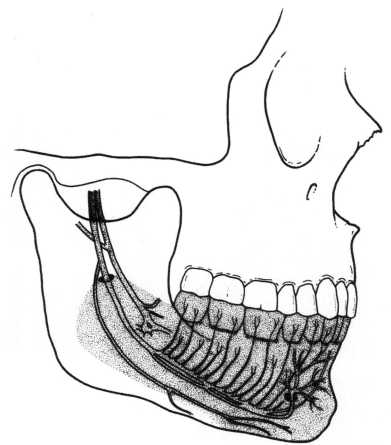

Figure 4.4b

quietly positive attitude by the dentist about a proposed injection of local anaesthetic instils confidence in the patient. Explanations of what is to happen in the dental procedure should include the local anaesthetic, so that the patient is aware of the nature of the treatment and is therefore in a position to give informed consent (see Chapter 11). In general, the more patients know about their treatment, the less they are frightened by it; fear of the unknown is commonly the source of unnecessary anxiety.

For anxious patients in need of reassurance, nothing builds confidence more than the experience of painless dental treatment, and successful local anaesthesia is the keystone of this principle. Every item of treatment completed gives the patient positive feedback and encouragement to face the next procedure. Therefore simple, achievable treatment goals should be tackled first, including selecting the areas of the mouth, such as the posterior maxilla, where local anaesthetics are routinely successful and easy to administer.

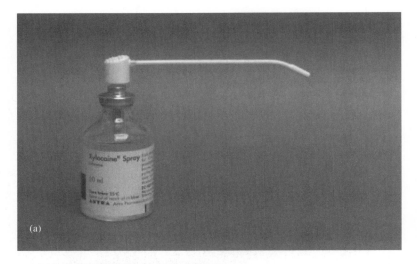

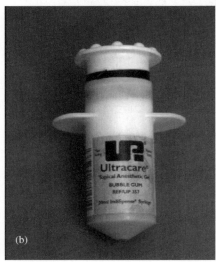

Figure 4.5.   A photograph of topical anaesthetic in (a) spray form or (b) flavoured paste. The spray is applied directly (c), the paste via a cotton wool roll (d).

The patient should be positioned comfortably in the chair, which is also adjusted to allow optimal access for the operator to the injection site. It is important that a clear view with unimpeded access to the relevant part of the mouth is maintained during the injection procedure. In order to achieve this both patient and operator should be as comfortable and relaxed as possible in the circumstances, with the patient receiving reassurance as necessary.

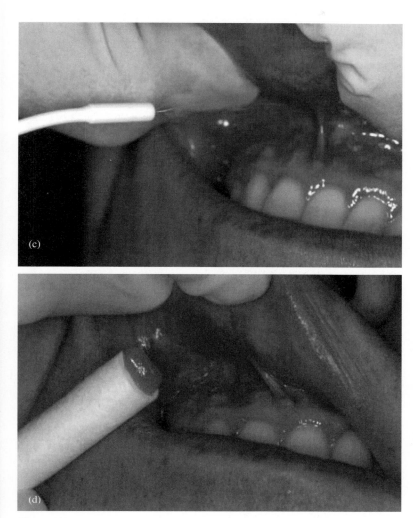

Figure 4.5

Surface anaesthesia

The aspect of local anaesthesia that most patients dread is the initial perforation of the tissues by the needle. Modern needles for dental local anaesthesia are extremely fine (27 or 30 gauge) and have sharp bevelled tips designed to facilitate atraumatic entry into the tissues, so minimising discomfort. Despite this, there are some areas in the mouth, particularly anteriorly in the labial sulci, where needle entry can be painful. The use of topical local anaesthetic supplied as a liquid spray or paste can eliminate this unpleasant sensation (Figure 4.5).

Minimizing the discomfort of needle entry can also be achieved in other ways:

- avoid brandishing the syringe and needle in front of the patient
- do not theatrically hide the syringe behind your back (some patients benefit from seeing how small the needle really is!)
- select the appropriate needle for the injection site – a finer gauge needle provokes less discomfort
- hold the mucosa taut but not stretched at the proposed injection site (Figure 4.6)
- for injections into the palate, a few seconds of gentle but increasing pressure exactly at the proposed injection site with the end of a dental mirror handle, just before placing the needle, modifies sensory input so eliminating the sharp sensation
- distract the patient's attention at the instant of injection with some comment on a subject that may appeal to the particular patient – but avoid asking questions that invite an answer!

Injecting the local anaesthetic solution

The most painful part of dental injections is the placement of the anaesthetic solution into the tissues once the needle is in place. This effect can be minimised in the following ways:

- warm the cartridges of local anaesthetic to 37° Centigrade – injecting cold solution is **very painful**
- inject the solution **slowly** – it is the distension of the tissues that causes the pain
- inject a small amount of anaesthetic solution (a few drops) just below the surface of the mucosa and wait 10–15 seconds before advancing the needle into the desired position for placement of the bulk of the solution
- avoid injecting the solution subperiosteally.

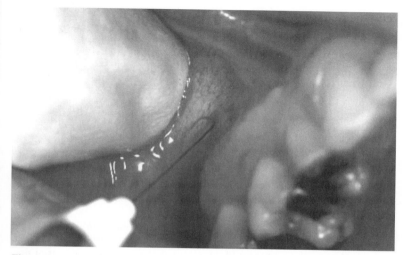

Figure 4.6.   The soft tissues are retracted and gently stretched to facilitate perforation of the mucosa by the needle.

Waiting sufficient time for anaesthesia

To be effective in achieving adequate anaesthesia, the local anaesthetic solution must diffuse either into the tissues to be anaesthetised in the case of an infiltration injection, or into the relevant nerve trunk for regional block anaesthesia. In either case the effect is not instantaneous and anaesthesia of sufficient depth to permit pain-free dental surgery normally takes about 5 minutes to be established, although the timing may vary considerably. Occasionally a regional block injection placed very close to the target nerve begins to take effect in seconds; with less accurate injections the anaesthetic solution must first diffuse through the tissues to reach the nerve, thus delaying the onset of anaesthesia. In cases where the solution must penetrate deep into the tissues to be effective, e.g. into the deep aspect of a periapical granuloma associated with a tooth for apicectomy, there may be a delay of several minutes. Allowing insufficient time before starting to operate is inviting the patient to perceive that the local anaesthetic has failed; a concept that may then be difficult to erase.

Testing for anaesthesia

As the local anaesthetic begins to take effect, the patient is able to report altered sensation of the soft tissues that usually accompanies dental anaesthesia. Asking the patient to describe the sensation indicates the level of anaethesia. The operator should distinguish between tingling of the tissue and complete numbness. While tingling of the lip or tongue may be the initial effect most noticeable to the patient, this does not signify that the pulps of the teeth are fully anaesthetised, as these structures take time to achieve adequate surgical anaesthesia.

Objective testing of the gingivae adjacent to the relevant tooth by gentle challenge with the point of a dental probe may give an indication that the periodontal tissues have been anaesthetised. When a tooth is to be extracted, firm pressure with a probe in the periodontal ligament is a more stringent test of anaesthesia, but these tests cannot indicate whether the dental pulp is anaesthetised. Sometimes a pulpitic tooth remains tender to percussion, suggesting that the pulp is not fully anaesthetised even when all the periodontal tissues are (see Chapter 7).

After achieving anaesthesia, an explanation of what the patient can expect from the local anaesthetic can usefully be reinforced at this stage. Sensations of pain and discomfort from the immediate surgical site should be eliminated by blockade of the sensory nerves supplying those structures. However, there is likely to be a feeling of pressure transmitted from the surgical site to unanaesthetised adjacent areas. It is important that the patient realises that these pressure sensations are not signs that the local anaesthetic has failed. It also helps to explain to the patient why some tissues are affected by the anaesthetic but others are not; for example the inferior dental nerve block does not anaesthetise the mucosa buccal to the molars.

Perhaps the definitive test of local anaesthetic success is whether the dental procedure can be carried out without discomfort to the patient. With this in mind, patients will be reassured to know that they can signal to the operator by raising a hand if the procedure causes them pain or discomfort.

Chapter 5

Maxillary anaesthesia

Maxillary teeth are normally easy to anaesthetise. The cortical bone of the maxilla is thin on its buccal aspect and local anaesthetic solution readily diffuses through it. As a consequence, the sensory nerves running through the maxilla and supplying both the pulps of the teeth and the surrounding alveolar bone are accessible to local anaesthetic placed in the buccal soft tissues adjacent to the target tooth using the technique of local infiltration. Satisfactory anaesthesia for most restorative procedures that require pulpal anaesthesia can be achieved with a single buccal infiltration injection, which of course also anaesthetises the buccal soft tissues. Dental extractions and other procedures encroaching on the palatal soft tissues require additional anaesthetic to be injected into the palate, as these tissues have a separate nerve supply.

Anaesthesia for restorative procedures in maxillary teeth

The maxillary teeth receive their sensory nerve supply from the anterior, middle and posterior superior alveolar (syn: dental) nerves (Figure 5.1), which are all branches of the maxillary division of the trigeminal nerve (see Glossary). Anaesthetising these nerves is readily achieved by blocking the peripheral fibres near where they enter the apical foramina of the teeth, using the technique of local infiltration.

The placement of 0.5–1.0 ml of local anaesthetic solution in the sulcus adjacent to the tooth requiring anaesthesia is relatively straightforward, and rarely fails (some precautions and modifications due to variation of local anatomy are considered later). For this reason, infiltration anaesthesia for maxillary teeth is a good starting point for the inexperienced student.

Standard technique

The tissues are retracted using a gloved finger and gently stretched, allowing easier penetration of the needle tip. A short needle (length

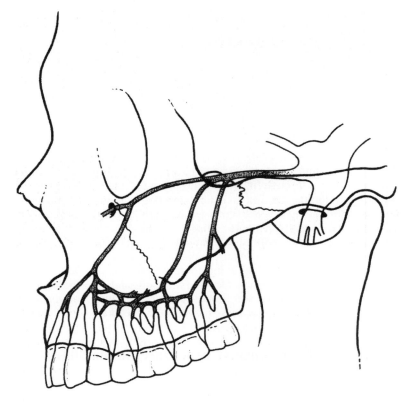

Figure 5.1.   Diagram to show the distribution of the maxillary division of the
trigeminal nerve into the anterior, middle and posterior branches.

20 mm, diameter 0.3 mm) is adequate to reach most injection sites in
the maxilla. The needle is placed so that the bevel of the end of the
needle faces the alveolar bone, and is advanced 1 mm into the soft
tissues (Figure 5.2). At this stage 3–4 drops of solution are deposited
into the mucosa, 10–15 seconds allowed for this to work and the needle
advanced to its correct depth just above the periosteum.

It is not necessary to contact bone. The anaesthetic solution should be
injected supra-periosteally; placing it under the periosteal layer, which
is richly innervated, causes a lot of pain.

By gently depressing the plunger of a modern aspirating syringe it is
possible to establish if any blood is aspirated into the cartridge. If this
is the case the needle position should be changed within the tissues, and

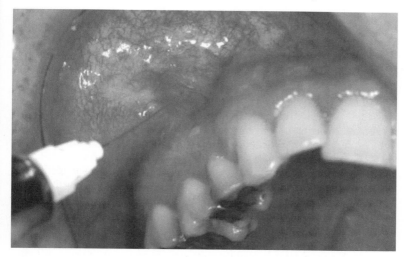

Figure 5.2.   Photograph of an infiltration injection into a premolar injection.

aspiration repeated to prevent the risk of intravascular injection. At this stage the main dose of anaesthetic (0.5–1.0 ml) is deposited into the tissues at a slow rate that does not unduly distend the soft tissues. Pressure is removed from the plunger and the needle is then withdrawn. The area may then be massaged with a gloved finger to assist diffusion of the anaesthetic solution.

Variation of procedures of infiltration for specific teeth

Central and lateral incisors
Infiltration anaesthesia should be given in the sulcus adjacent to the tooth in question. Placement of anaesthetic solution at the anterior aspect of the mouth can be very painful; therefore surface anaesthesia, the use of a fine needle (0.3 mm diameter), and slow injection of the solution are necessary to reduce patient discomfort.

Canine teeth
Enter the tissues near the apex of the lateral incisor or the first premolar. The tissues may be more easily accessible here than directly over the canine eminence, and this allows a relatively comfortable injection.

Premolar teeth
These teeth are normally easy to anaesthetise using the standard infiltration technique.

First molar teeth
The mesial root is usually supplied by the middle superior alveolar dental nerve, while the distal and palatal roots are supplied by the posterior superior alveolar dental nerve. In this region the dense zygomatic buttress joins the maxilla, and may present a barrier to infiltration directly buccal to the first molar. Where difficulty is encountered, anaesthesia may be achieved by placing 0.5 ml of solution anterior to the zygomatic buttress, often near the premolar teeth, and also 1.0 ml distal to the zygomatic arch to complete the anaesthesia.

Second and third molar teeth
Anaesthesia is performed by placing 1.0 ml of solution distal to the zygomatic buttress. Care must be taken not to place the needle too deep into the tissues where it could encounter the pterygoid venous plexus; as a result the anaesthetic solution could be injected intravenously. Also, damaging the plexus might cause bleeding into the tissues and result in formation of a haematoma.

Summary of maxillary infiltration
1. Gently stretch the mucosa by retracting the lip or cheek
2. Apply surface anaesthetic if appropriate
3. Puncture the mucosa with the bevel of the needle facing the bone opposite the tooth in question
4. Place 4–5 drops of solution within 1 mm of the mucosal surface
5. Wait 10–15 seconds, advance the needle 0.5–1.0 cm and aspirate to ensure that a blood vessel has not been entered (if blood were apparent, the needle would need to be re-sited)
6. Place 0.5–1.0 ml of solution supra-periosteally
7. Withdraw the needle carefully
8. Massage the mucosa to enhance diffusion of the solution, if required
9. Allow at least 5 minutes before treatment is commenced.

Anaesthesia for surgical treatment and restorative procedures involving soft tissues of the palate

The buccal and labial soft tissues are anaesthetised by buccal/labial infiltration. It is not possible to anaesthetise the hard and soft palate by this approach. These tissues require separate soft tissue injections directly into the palate. In general, the soft tissues of the hard palate are tightly bound down to the underlying bone especially near the gingival margins of the teeth and in the midline. Placement of solution in these regions can be very painful. About halfway between the midline and the palatal aspect of the teeth is a zone with slightly thicker submucosa through which the vessels and nerves supplying the palate run (Figure 5.3a, b). It is here that the needle should enter the tissues for two

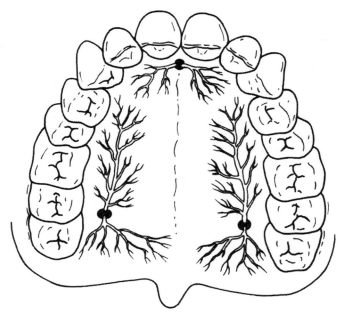

Figure 5.3a.   Diagram to illustrate the position of the nerves supplying the palate.

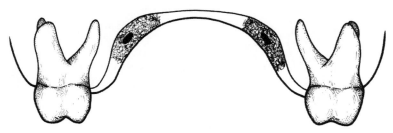

Figure 5.3b.   Coronal section through the palate in the region of the first molars showing the position of the nerves and vessels within the palatal soft tissues.

reasons: to place the local anaesthetic solution close to the branches of the palatine nerves, and because injection at this site is much less uncomfortable.

Greater and lesser palatine nerves

These nerves are sensory to the soft tissues palatal to the molars and premolars, and they leave the palate via their respective foramina (Figure 5.3a). The lesser palatine nerves turn posteriorly to supply the mucosa overlying the soft palate, while the greater palatine nerve passes forwards and supplies the mucosa overlying the hard palate as far anteriorly as the canine tooth. Beyond this the palatal mucosa of the premaxilla is supplied by the incisive nerve. The precise boundary between the territories of these two nerves is, however, variable. The technique of injection for the palate is to introduce a fine needle at right angles to the surface of the mucosa halfway between the midline and the gingival margin of the tooth to be anaesthetised. Only a few drops of solution can be injected into the tight tissue compartment without

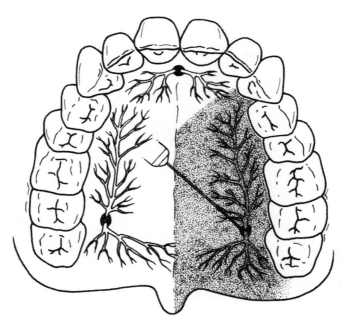

Figure 5.4.   Diagram showing the area of anaesthesia achieved when the greater palatine nerves are blocked at the foramen.

causing undue tension in the tissues and the attendant unnecessary discomfort. The greater palatine nerve can also be blocked at the foramen (Figure 5.3a) when the area of anaesthesia depicted in Figure 5.4 is achieved. The anterior boundary of this area varies with overlap from the incisive nerve and can be as far back as the premolar region. Anaesthesia of the soft palate may also occur as the lesser palatine nerves are often blocked as well; this is not dangerous but may be an unpleasant sensation for the patient.

Incisive nerve

This nerve is a terminal branch of the naso-palatine nerve (long spheno-palatine) and supplies sensation to the soft tissues palatal to the incisors. It leaves the bony palate by the incisive canal just behind the incisive papilla. The best site to anaesthetise the incisive nerve is directly over the incisive foramen (Figure 5.3a). As with the injections further back in the palate, the tight muco-periosteal tissue will only accommodate a few drops of anaesthetic solution. Figure 5.5 shows the area anaesthetised, but note that there is variation in the boundary between the incisive and greater palatine nerve territories.

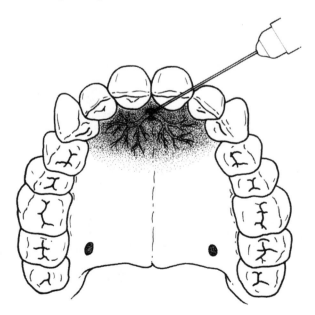

Figure 5.5. Diagram showing the area of anaesthesia achieved when the incisive nerve is blocked at the foramen.

The combination of a greater palatine block and an incisive block produces anaesthesia of the whole of one side of the palate. This combination would be suitable for the extraction of several teeth in that quadrant of the mouth.

Anaesthetising the palatal tissues with minimal discomfort

In this technique the standard buccal infiltration is given and the tissues allowed to become anaesthetised. Then, using the same needle, the interdental papillae by the tooth in question are anaesthetised by direct injection into each papilla from the buccal side. Only small volumes of solution are needed and the solution is placed very superficially. After 5–10 seconds the needle is advanced between the teeth 2–3 mm and 4–5 drops of solution deposited, 5–10 seconds are then allowed for diffusion, after which the needle tip is advanced towards the palate (Figure 5.6). This continues until the solution can be seen blanching the palatal aspect of the mucosa and papilla, but the needle must not perforate the palatal mucosa.

At this stage 3–4 drops of solution are placed, the needle is withdrawn completely from the tissues and the papilla on the other side of the tooth is anaesthetised in the same way. The palatal mucosa can

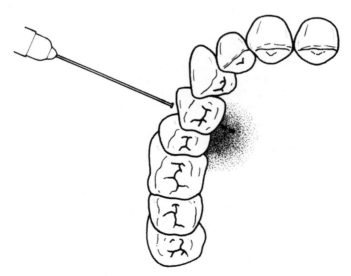

Figure 5.6.   Diagram showing an intra-papillary injection extended into the palatal tissues between the teeth.

then be injected as described above, and it is usually sufficiently anaes-thetised so that no discomfort is felt by the patient. Another technique is to apply steady, firm pressure to the intended injection site in the palate for several seconds using a dental mirror handle. Introduction of the needle at precisely the same place is then disguised by this 'counter irritant' procedure.

Summary of technique for anaesthesia of a maxillary first premolar for extraction

1. Place buccal infiltration 0.5–1.0 ml in the sulcus adjacent to the first premolar
2. After 2 minutes infiltrate the mesial papilla of first premolar stopping just short of palatal mucosa
3. Anaesthetise the distal papilla of first premolar
4. Place 0.2 ml of solution in palate opposite first premolar between midline and gingival margin.

Infra-orbital nerve block

Anterior superior alveolar nerve block
Due to the success of standard infiltration anaesthetics in the maxilla, block anaesthesia is seldom necessary. Occasionally a wider field of anaesthesia extending over the anterior maxilla is required. Blockade of the infra-orbital nerve at its foramen also includes branches of the anterior superior alveolar nerve. This results in anaesthesia of both hard and soft tissues of the anterior maxilla and upper lip.

The infra-orbital foramen lies just below the inferior orbital margin about halfway along its length and is often palpable through the skin (Figure 5.7a). The infra-orbital nerve (a terminal branch of the maxillary nerve) is easily approached from the upper labial sulcus opposite the canine tooth. Use of a long needle (35 mm) is necessary to achieve adequate depth safely (Figure 5.7b). From the entry point in the sulcus the needle tip is directed towards a finger placed over the infra-orbital foramen, injecting small quantities of solution as the needle is slowly advanced. When the needle tip is in place over the foramen, the palpating finger can detect the slight distension of the tissue and 1–2 ml of solution are injected (Figure 5.7c). The area of anaesthesia involving the anterior maxilla is also shown in Figure 5.7.

Provision of infiltration anaesthesia for multiple adjacent teeth

In these cases a long needle is used and rather than injecting separately in multiple areas, the needle is advanced within the tissues parallel to

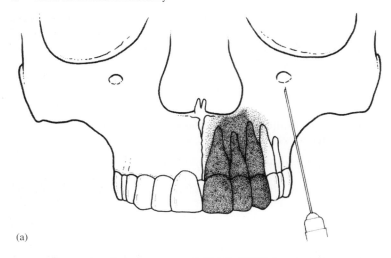

(a)

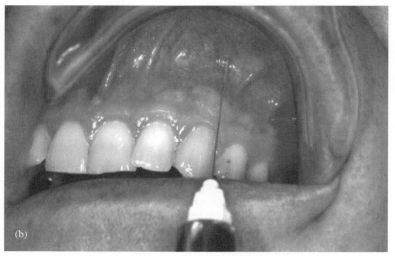

(b)

Figure 5.7. (a) Diagram showing blocking of the infra-orbital nerve at the foramen and the resultant area of anaesthesia of the teeth and surrounding bone. (b) A photograph showing the use of a long needle to place the solution close to the infra-orbital foramen and (c) the use of a finger to palpate the notch in the infra-orbital ridge.

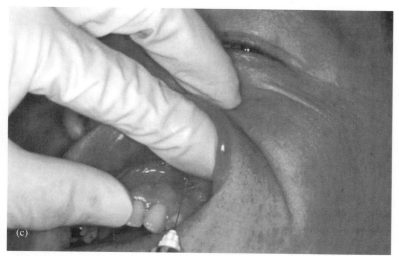

Figure 5.7

the occlusal plane, commencing at the most anterior teeth. In this way the area of anaesthesia is slowly enlarged.

Further reading

Agur, A. M. R. (ed) (1991). *Grant's Atlas of Anatomy,* 9th edition. Williams and Wilkins.
McMinn, R. M. H. (1994). *Anatomy Regional and Applied,* 9th edition. Churchill Livingstone.

Chapter 6

Mandibular anaesthesia

The key to successful local anaesthesia is to put the right amount of local anaesthetic solution in the right place and wait for the correct length of time for it to work. This is especially true for the regional block technique needed to anaesthetise the inferior dental nerve. Knowing where to place the injection is the difficult part and requires some basic knowledge and understanding of the local anatomy, the structures to be anaesthetised and their sensory nerve supply.

The cortical bone over most of the mandibular body is too thick to permit penetration of the local anaesthetic solution from buccal infiltration and so the inferior dental nerve is normally anaesthetised more proximally at the mandibular foramen.

Most local anaesthetic injections in the mouth are intended to anaesthetise the pulps of teeth so that restorative procedures can be carried out painlessly. Extraction of teeth and surgery involving their surrounding tissues dictate that anaesthesia should also encompass the periodontal tissues, both hard and soft. Less frequently anaesthesia of the tongue, lips or cheeks may be needed for a variety of soft tissue surgery including biopsy or excision of small swellings. The pattern of anaesthesia required therefore varies with the restorative or surgical task. In general, the types of anaesthesia and operative procedures are detailed in Table 6.1.

Anaesthesia for restorative procedures in mandibular teeth

All of the lower teeth receive their sensory nerve supply from the inferior dental nerve (syn: inferior alveolar nerve – see Glossary), a branch of the mandibular division of the trigeminal nerve. Anaesthetising the inferior dental nerve in the adult jaw involves blocking the nerve trunk before it enters the bone at the mandibular foramen on the medial aspect of the ramus, just behind the lingula. Further anteriorly the nerve runs within the dense bone of the mandible and is not readily accessible to local anaesthetic solution until it exits

Table 6.1   Combinations of local anaesthetic injections required for multiple sites in the mandible

Procedure to be undertaken and area to be anaesthetised	Nerves to be anaesthetised
Restorative procedures on teeth from 8 to 2 Extraction of lower 4 3 2	Inferior dental block (+ lingual, which is achieved with the same injection)
Extraction of 8 7 6 5	Inferior dental block (with lingual nerve block as above) + long buccal nerve anaesthesia
Restorative procedures on 1 2	Labial infiltration opposite the lower incisor (to anaesthetise the branches of the mental and incisive nerve)
Extraction of 1 2	Labial infiltration as above plus infiltration lingually opposite the lower central incisor to anaesthetise branches of the lingual nerve; or bilateral mental (incisive nerve) block + lingual infiltration, as above
Restorative procedures on 4 3 2	Mental (incisive nerve) block
Extraction of 4 3 2	Mental nerve block as above plus lingual infiltration to anaesthetise branches of the lingual nerve. Advantage of mental block over inferior dental block is the restricted area of anaesthesia and the absence of tongue numbness, as the lingual nerve not is blocked at the same time. The disadvantage of mental block is that anaesthesia is less reliable

from the mental foramen on the buccal aspect of the mandible, in the premolar region.

The placement of local anaesthetic solution at the mental foramen will anaesthetise the mental nerve to give soft tissue numbness of the labial gingivae, the lower lip and chin. The anaesthetic solution will also diffuse via the mental foramen to reach the incisive branch which supplies the pulps of lower teeth from the first premolar forwards to the midline where there is some cross-over of the nerve supply from the opposite side. The incisive nerve may also be anaesthetised by buccal infiltration in the lower incisor region due to the thin buccal cortex of bone at this site.

The inferior dental nerve block

The distribution of anaesthesia provided by the inferior dental (ID) block is shown in Figure 6.1a, b. It includes the bone of the mandibular body and the pulps of all of the teeth on that side of the mouth, except perhaps the central incisor where there may be some cross-over supply from the inferior dental nerve on the opposite side.

The injection is given with a long dental needle (35 mm) in a standard aspirating cartridge syringe. Careful positioning of the patient in the chair should permit comfort for the patient and clear access to the injection site for the operator. There is no correct position to adopt, as the landmarks for correct placement of the injection solution relate to the patient's anatomy and not to some arbitrary vertical or horizontal plane.

The key points of the local anatomy are set out in the Figures 6.1a, 6.2 and 6.3. The operator must realise that the target nerve runs through the infra-temporal fossa between the base of the skull at the foramen ovale and the mandibular foramen. The nerve is accessible to local

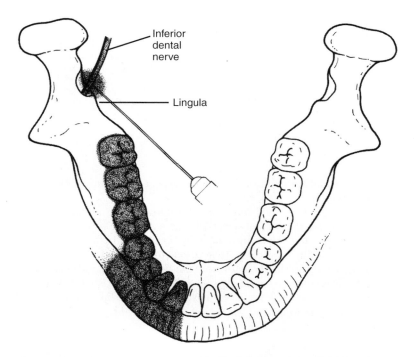

Figure 6.1.a.   Diagram showing inferior dental block anaesthesia of all the mandibular teeth on the right side of the mandible and the buccal gingivae of the lower first premolar to the lateral incisor. In addition the soft tissues of the lower lip on the right are anaesthetised.

anaesthetic solution anywhere in its passage through this anatomical space, but it is routinely blocked at the mandibular foramen, just behind the lingula.

It is vital to appreciate the position of this foramen and unfortunately it is somewhat variable. Normally it lies at a point halfway between the maximum concavity of the coronoid notch on the anterior surface of the ramus of the mandible and the maximum concavity of the posterior border of the ramus. Both of these two points can readily be palpated in the living patient as well as on a dried skull (Figure 6.4). The index finger and thumb of one hand should palpate these important landmarks while the injection is given. The aim is to place the needle tip against bone halfway between thumb and finger tip; there is a high success rate if the anaesthetic solution is injected in this position.

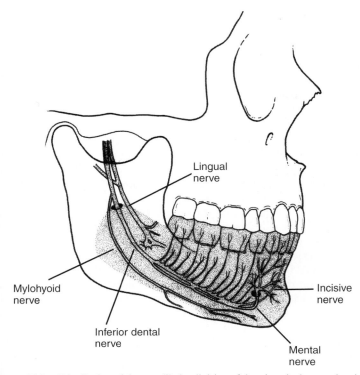

Figure 6.1.b.   Distribution of the mandibular division of the trigeminal nerve showing the branches anaesthetised when an inferior dental block is given. These include the lingual nerve and the mylohyoid branch of the inferior dental nerve. The diagram shows only the hard tissue distribution of anaesthesia.

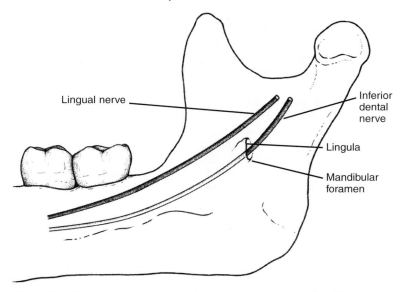

Figure 6.2. Medial view of the mandibular ramus showing the position of the lingula and mandibular foramen.

The needle should enter the tissues at the back of the mouth just medial to the border of the ramus of the mandible, at a level halfway up the thumb, which is palpating the coronoid notch. The barrel of the syringe should be parallel to the occlusal plane of the lower teeth, and under normal circumstances in the dentate patient this will make the point of entry of the needle just above the occlusal level of the last standing molar tooth. Another landmark, often quoted as being useful but not easily identified, is the pterygomandibular raphe. This fibrous structure, which separates the buccinator from the superior constrictor muscle, runs from the pterygoid hamulus down to a point on the mandible in the retromolar region. It raises a ridge of mucous membrane, which forms a 'V' shape with the anterior border of the mandible. The needle for the ID block passes lateral to the pterygo-mandibular raphe and medial to the ramus of the mandible, i.e. within the limbs of this 'V' (Figure 6.5).

Having penetrated the tissues for a depth of approximately 1 cm, the needle is turned a little more laterally by moving the barrel of the syringe across the midline to the opposite premolar or molar region. The needle is then advanced further until bony contact is made on the medial aspect of the mandible. The reader must appreciate that the ramus of the mandible flares laterally away from the advancing needle and, moreover, this angle increases behind the lingula (Figure 6.5). Therefore, the operator should aim to touch the bone with the needle tip at or just in front of the lingula and then 'walk' the needle gently backwards keeping intermittent contact with the bone until no further bony contact is felt. The needle should now be just behind the lingula, where the mandibular ramus flares laterally. Assuming that the needle is at the correct vertical position then its tip should now be precisely over the mandibular foramen.

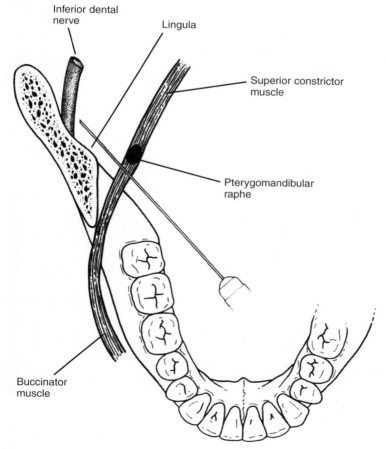

Inferior dental
nerve

Lingula

Superior constrictor
muscle

Pterygomandibular
raphe

Buccinator
muscle

Figure 6.3.   Horizontal section in the mandibular occlusal plane showing the pterygomandibular raphe; the injection site is lateral to this landmark.

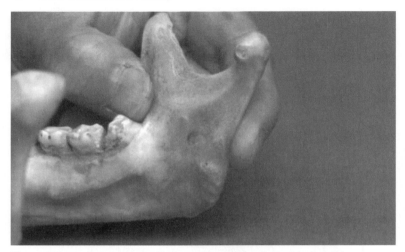

Figure 6.4.   A photograph of a dried mandible showing the positioning of the palpating finger and thumb in the concavities of the ramus anteriorly and posteriorly. The mandibular foramen is found midway between the tips of the finger and thumb.

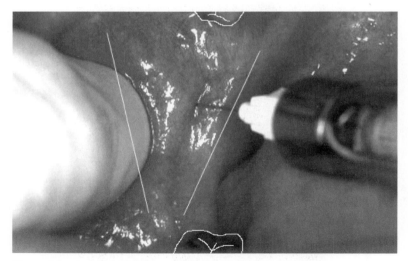

Figure 6.5.   An intra-oral photograph showing the medial position of the pterygomandibular raphe. At the bottom edge of the photograph, the occlusal surface of the last molar can be seen. The medial line represents the angulation of the pterygomandibular raphe, while the gloved thumb is palpating the anterior aspect of the ascending ramus of the mandible. The lateral line represents the ascending ramus. These two structures make a 'V' which makes the ideal entry point for the needle.

Following aspiration to guard against intravascular injection, the placement of 2.0 ml of anaesthetic solution should therefore result in a satisfactory block of the inferior dental nerve. If bone is contacted prematurely then the needle can be advanced further posteriorly. If the bone cannot be contacted, the needle is probably too far back and should be withdrawn slightly and then re-angled further laterally towards the ramus. Bone contact with the needle is made with very light pressure to avoid damage to the fine point of the needle tip. Figure 6.6 shows a needle tip bent into a hook by clumsy bone contact.

An accurate injection works rapidly; most injections start to have some effect within a few minutes. Occasionally it takes longer. The first sign of success is normally some tingling along the lateral aspect of the tongue. This injection blocks the lingual nerve in a very high proportion of patients. Tingling of the lower lip (supplied by the mental nerve which is a branch of the inferior dental) is usually appreciated a short time afterwards. If there is no change of sensation in the lower lip within 5 minutes then the block is unlikely to work. The tingling sensation is slowly replaced by a total absence of sensation and at this

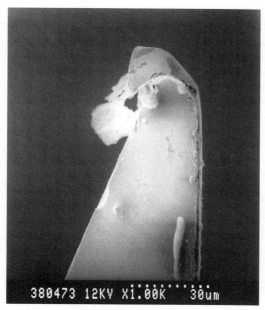

Figure 6.6.   A scanning electron micrograph showing the tip of a needle bent to form a 'hook' following inadvertent bony contact.

point the pulps of the teeth should also be anaesthetised. Note that pulpal anaesthesia is not normally achieved whilst the lower lip is in its 'tingling' phase.

Practical problems in giving an inferior dental block
- The patient needs to keep his/her mouth open wide during the administration of the standard inferior dental block. If the patient closes his/her mouth even partially, then the needle may pass too far inferiorly and miss the mandibular foramen. Placement of the local anaesthetic solution at this point does not reach the inferior dental nerve because the nerve is contained within the mandible at this level. Note that it is better to be too high with placement of the solution than too low.
- Placement of the needle too far back may result in losing the landmark on the ramus of the mandible as the needle is advanced. If bony contact cannot be achieved then the needle is probably too posterior. Injection of solution at this site does not find the inferior dental nerve but may find the facial nerve, as the needle tip may have passed into the capsule of the parotid gland. The patient then suffers temporary paralysis of the side of the face.
- The patient's tongue may obstruct the desired point of entry into the tissues, or the patient may retch when the instrument is positioned towards the back of the mouth. The use of surface anaesthesia and reassurance should overcome both these problems.
- The position of the mandibular foramen may vary and this can give rise to difficulty in achieving anaesthesia, particularly if the foramen is high up the ramus. This anatomical variation can readily be spotted on a dental panoramic tomograph (DPT) if available.
- The position of the mandibular foramen appears to change with age. In the young child the ramus is not fully developed and the foramen is low down, at or below the occlusal level of the lower teeth. In the dentate adult the foramen is at or just above the occlusal level of the lower teeth. However, in the partially dentate, particularly elderly patients with missing molar teeth, the foramen is very much higher than the level of the remaining alveolus, which is well below the original occlusal level of the teeth (Figure 6.7a, b).

Mental block (incisive block)

A limited area of anaesthesia in the anterior aspect of the mandible may be achieved by placing approximately 1.0 ml of local anaesthetic solution adjacent to the mental foramen. Although called a mental block, the aim of this injection is normally to anaesthetise the incisive branch of the inferior dental nerve which supplies the pulps of the teeth anterior to the mental foramen, namely the lower first premolar, canine and incisor teeth. The area of anaesthesia achieved is shown in Figure 6.8.

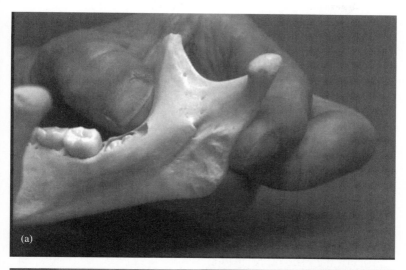

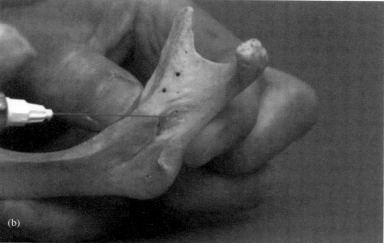

Figure 6.7.   The mandible of both a child (a) and an edentulous patient (b) shown with a long needle in position to place the solution close to the mandibular foramen. The anterior and posterior concavities of the ramus, shown in Figure 6.3, still indicate the level of the mandibular foramen.

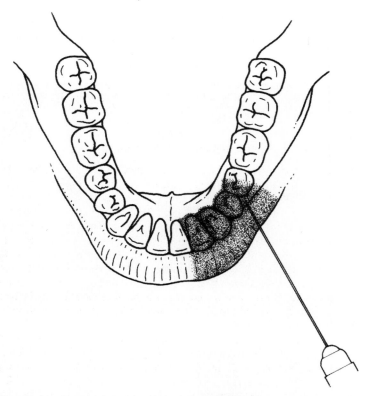

Figure 6.8.   Mental block anaesthesia. The area of anaesthesia is shown following injection over the mental foramen (between the apices of the premolar teeth).

The position of the mental foramen is normally just below and between the apices of the lower premolar teeth. Its precise position may vary between individuals and can usually be easily located on a DPT radiograph if available. The foramen is best approached with the anaesthetic needle from a superior direction. The soft tissues should be punctured in the depth of the sulcus and the needle inserted to just beyond where the apices of the lower premolar teeth are estimated to be. It is helpful to touch the surface of the bone gently with the needle to ensure that the anaesthetic solution is placed close to the foramen, but no attempt should be made to gain access to the foramen with the tip of the needle in case the mental nerve is traumatised directly. Normally, 1.0 ml of anaesthetic solution is sufficient to induce rapid and complete anaesthesia.

Anaesthesia of incisor teeth

In the incisor region the labial cortex of the mandible is thin even in an adult. This will allow sufficient local anaesthetic solution to diffuse through and anaesthetise the pulps of the teeth.

The procedure is very similar to that used for the maxilla, injecting 0.5 ml at the depth of the labial sulcus and opposite the tooth to be treated.

Restorative procedures in children (Rule of 10)

The mandibular bone in children has a cortex which is much less dense than that in the adult. As a result, buccal infiltration injections placed directly opposite the tooth for restoration may adequately penetrate the bone and give satisfactory pulpal anaesthesia as an alternative to an ID block; but it must be stressed that the situation in individual patients may vary. For practical purposes this technique is successful only in the deciduous dentition of young children, and as a general guide a 'Rule of 10' has been described. In this technique each tooth is allocated a score: A = 1, B = 2, C = 3, D = 4 and E = 5. The most distal tooth to be restored is added to the child's age rounded to the nearest year. If this is 10 and above an inferior dental block is indicated; below 10 an infiltration is all that is necessary.

For example if a child presents at age 5 years 11 months (rounded up to 6), with a deciduous second primary molar (scoring 5) requiring restoration, the score is 11 and an inferior dental block is indicated. If a child presents aged 4 years 1 month (rounded to 4), and a deciduous first primary molar (D scoring 4) is to be restored, the total is 8 and an infiltration is appropriate.

Procedures requiring anaesthesia of the surrounding gingivae and soft tissues

Some procedures may involve encroaching on the soft tissues around the tooth, e.g. the placement of a matrix band in a deep position. The surrounding gingivae may not have been anaesthetised by the inferior dental block (see the extent of anaesthesia obtained with an ID block, as shown in Figure 6.1a). The gingivae may easily be anaesthetised by the placement of a small amount of local anaesthetic directly at the site involved, either by an infiltration injection in the sulcus or an intra-papillary injection (see Chapter 5). More extensive soft tissue periodontal procedures may require a blockade of other sensory branches of the trigeminal nerve, e.g. the lingual and long buccal nerves (see next section).

The extraction of teeth and other dental procedures requiring soft tissue anaesthesia around the teeth usually necessitate more than one injection, as often more than the inferior dental nerve distribution is involved.

Long buccal nerve

This nerve is a branch of the mandibular nerve and is given off high in the infra-temporal fossa. It passes downwards and forwards winding around the anterior border of the ramus of the mandible in the coronoid notch, passing laterally out into the cheek tissues and down towards the buccal sulcus in the lower molar region. It supplies the buccal gingivae and the vestibular mucosa from the retromolar region as far forward as the second premolar. The area of mucosa supplied by the long buccal nerve is shown (Figure 6.9).

Although the nerve is described as having a main trunk through its intra-oral course, it often runs as a plexus of small branches into the buccal tissues. The nerve can therefore be blocked by an injection of anaesthetic solution as it crosses the anterior border of the ramus distal to the third molars, where 0.5–1 ml of solution should be adequate. Its terminal branches are also accessible to an infiltration injection close to the target tooth. Anaesthesia of this nerve rarely fails.

The lingual nerve

The lingual nerve is almost always blocked adequately when an inferior dental block injection is given. The lingual nerve runs anterior to the inferior alveolar nerve on a parallel course down through the infratemporal fossa and passes close to the anterior part of the medial aspect of the ramus (Figure 6.2). From there it passes close to, or in contact with the periosteum of the mandible in the third molar region just above the mylohyoid line, and gains access to the floor of the mouth, having a close relationship to the submandibular duct before passing into and innervating the tongue. It also gives branches to the floor of the mouth and the lingual gingivae of the same side of the mouth up to the midline.

For practical purposes, it is not necessary to give a separate injection to block the lingual nerve once an inferior dental block is in place. However, on occasions when an inferior alveolar block has not been used for an extraction (if a mental block to anaesthetise the incisive branch is given), then a separate infiltration of anaesthetic on the lingual aspect of the mandible will be required to block these branches of the lingual nerve. In this case the anaesthetic solution should be administered into the lax tissues of the floor of the mouth just below the

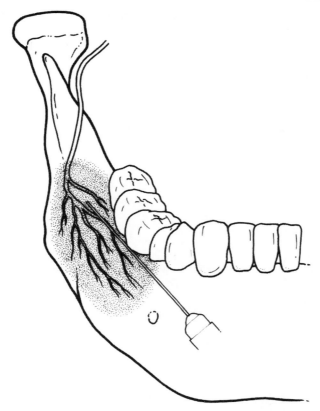

Figure 6.9.   Diagram illustrating the distribution of the long buccal nerve and the area of anaesthesia resulting from its blockade.

attached gingivae; 0.5 ml of solution is normally adequate and should be given at a point adjacent to the target tooth. The area supplied by the lingual nerve is shown in Figure 6.10.

Bilateral procedures in the mandible

Procedures can be undertaken bilaterally in the mandible using local anaesthesia. The combination of an inferior dental (and therefore lingual) block on one side and a mental (incisive) on the other, with or without lingual infiltration, will give an area of anaesthesia from the last molar tooth on the side of the inferior dental block around to the first premolar on the opposite side. A slightly more limited field of work on

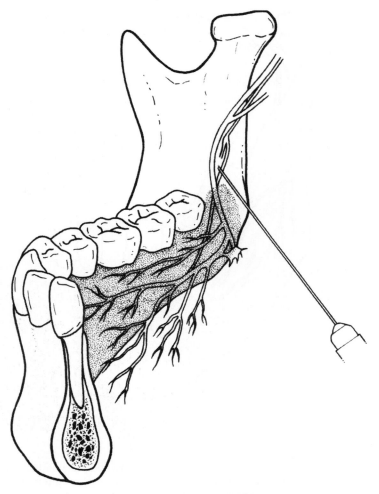

Figure 6.10.   Diagram illustrating the distribution of the lingual nerve and the site of regional block. The lingual nerve is usually anaesthetised when an inferior dental block is given.

the side opposite the inferior dental block can be achieved using labial and lingual infiltrations in the anterior mandible.

In certain circumstances it is useful to give bilateral inferior dental blocks. This permits surgery at the back of the mouth bilaterally (as in removing two lower third molar teeth).

In the authors' experience the placement of bilateral blocks is tolerated by the patient, and does not appear to embarrass the ability of the patient to defend the airway.

Aberrant nerve supply to the mandible and lower teeth

Occasionally, difficulty in anaesthetising the pulps of some lower teeth may be encountered even following successful blockade of the inferior dental nerve. This may result from some collateral sensory innervation running with either the mylohyoid branch of the inferior dental (which may be given off high above the mandibular foramen), the lingual nerve or the long buccal nerve. In each case infiltrating locally around the tooth in the area from which the collateral nerve supply is anticipated normally rectifies the problem. The anaesthetic solution may be placed as an infiltration close to the periosteum, via the intra-osseous route or alternatively as an intraligamentary injection (see Chapter 7).

Further reading

Curzon, M. E. J., Roberts, J. F. and Kennedy, D. B. (1991). *Paediatric Operative Dentistry*, 4th edition. Wright.

Management of the difficult case

Introduction

For most patients and most procedures, sufficient anaesthesia can be gained by infiltration and/or block anaesthesia of an adequate volume of anaesthetic solution in the appropriate place(s). However, there is a small group of patients who report frequent difficulty with achieving anaesthesia when a local anaesthetic is administered. Various reasons have been cited including poor technique, inadequate volume of anaesthetic solution, inflamed tissues at the site of injection, pulpal hyperaemia and abnormal anatomy. Generally speaking, giving a greater volume of anaesthetic at the correct site with supplemental injections achieves the desired effect. Alternative approaches have been proposed and these will now be considered.

Intraligamentary injection

The aim of this injection is to introduce local anaesthetic solution into the periodontal ligament of a tooth to achieve pulpal anaesthesia and to enable extraction of the tooth. The intention is to place the needle several millimetres into the periodontal ligament before injecting (Figure 7.1); in reality the solution escapes into the surrounding cancellous bone so it effectively is an intra-osseous injection. Normally 0.2 ml is injected; this volume is far in excess of that of the periodontal ligament space. It is usually effective in achieving anaesthesia, and has the advantage of anaesthetising a small area of the mouth, in contrast to an infiltration injection, so there is less associated soft tissue numbness.

Prior to injection the gingival sulcus should be disinfected by rubbing with a cotton bud soaked in a chlorhexidine mouthwash solution, to reduce bacterial inoculation into the bone. Surface anaesthetic should be applied to the gingival sulcus: the intraligamentary syringe is loaded with a standard anaesthetic cartridge and a special short fine needle. The needle is placed in the gingival crevice and introduced into the periodontal ligament for several millimetres. The lever on the syringe is

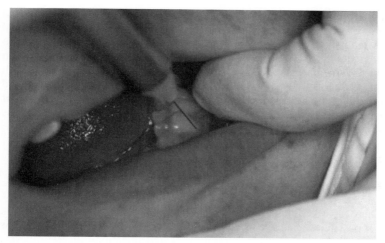

Figure 7.1. An intraligamentary injection in the region of the mandibular first premolar. The solution is placed in the periodontal ligament space.

then squeezed to inject 0.2 ml of the solution. It may be necessary to inject around each root of a multirooted tooth. Anaesthesia is normally achieved swiftly, but its duration is often limited to about 30 minutes using lignocaine with adrenaline. During this period there is virtually no blood flow in the pulp; techniques used on a vital tooth, during, for example, restorative procedures, should not further compromise this reduction in pulpal perfusion. It is important not to inject into infected tissues to prevent postoperative discomfort. There are rarely post-operative problems of significance, although the teeth can sometimes feel transiently displaced from the socket. Patients may complain of the same sensations as occur with a 'high' restoration.

Intra-osseous injection

This is now an outdated technique as it has been superseded by the intraligamentary injection. The technique consists of drilling a fine hole through the cortical plate of bone to allow an anaesthetic needle to be introduced into the cancellous bone close to the apex of the tooth to be anaesthetised. Ideally, before injection the mucosa should be disinfected with a chlorhexidine mouthwash solution, a surface anaesthetic applied and then a fine twist drill in a low-speed handpiece used to perforate the mucosa and cortical bone in an appropriate place. Care must be taken to avoid important structures such as underlying roots of teeth and neurovascular bundles. After making the opening through the cortical plate, a short needle on a standard syringe is inserted and the solution injected. Anaesthesia is normally achieved immediately and, as with intraligamentary anaesthesia, it is of short duration. There is a risk with this technique of injecting into a vascular channel within the bone, and therefore the adrenaline within the solution may cause a transient tachycardia. In patients with cardiac problems intra-osseous injections should be avoided.

Intrapulpal injection

There are occasions, particularly in teeth with acute pulpitis, when it is not possible to achieve effective pulpal anaesthesia using block and/or infiltration anaesthesia, even with repeated injections. In these cases, where the pulp is going to be extirpated or the tooth extracted, it may be possible to gain access to the partially anaesthetised pulp to insert a needle (Figure 7.2).

A small quantity is injected (< 0.1 ml); this rapidly achieves anaesthesia of approximately 10 minutes' duration, which is sufficient to allow the pulp to be extirpated with files. Patients are often aware of

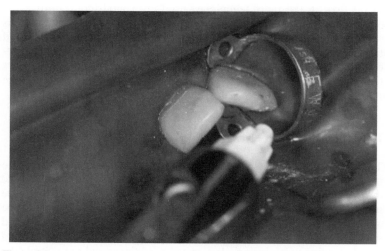

Figure 7.2.   An intrapulpal injection undertaken on a tooth isolated with rubber dam prior to pulp extirpation.

momentary unpleasantness as it is given, but are then relieved to be free of pain from a tooth which has probably been very uncomfortable.

Abnormal anatomy

When local anaesthesia is not achieved, the operator may consider that the problem is due to a variation in the normal pattern of nerve supply. It may be so in a small number of cases. On some occasions repeating the injection will be successful. In the case of difficult maxillary teeth, additional anaesthetic solution given palatally will usually achieve anaesthesia. A common problem affecting mandibular teeth is failure to achieve anaesthesia with a mandibular block injection; this may be because:

1. The solution has been placed in the wrong position (see Chapter 6)
2. The mandibular foramen on the medial aspect of the ascending ramus is higher than normal; its position may be observed on a DPT, if available
3. There is additional nerve supply to the mandibular molar teeth from a branch of the long buccal nerve; this can be corrected by buccal infiltration
4. There is additional nerve supply to the mandibular teeth from the mylohyoid nerve; this can be corrected by lingual infiltration.

These alternative techniques, used in conjunction with conventional regional block and infiltration anaesthesia, have been successful in all clinical circumstances in the authors' experience.

Further reading

Cohen, H. P., Cha, B. Y. and Spangberg, L. S. W. (1993). Endodontic anaesthesia in mandibular molars: a clinical study. *Journal of Endodontics*, **19**, 370–373.
Meechan, J. G. (1999). How to overcome failed local anaesthesia. *British Dental Journal*, **186**, 15–20.

Chapter 8

Selection of patients for treatment under local anaesthesia

The vast majority of dental procedures that require anaesthesia are undertaken with the use of local anaesthetic for the simple reason that, with very few exceptions, local anaesthesia is the safest, most effective and most convenient form of anaesthesia for dentistry.

General anaesthesia may be needed for certain types of treatment, e.g. complex surgery, or because of the patient's inability to co-operate with the treatment. However, general anaesthesia carries a higher risk of complications, some of them serious, both during the operative procedure and afterwards. It should therefore only be used when there are clear and specific indications.

Sedation administered either by the intravenous or the inhalational route, offers an effective and relatively safe way of assisting some patients to accept treatment under local anaesthesia, and raises the threshold for requiring a general anaesthetic.

The determinants of anaesthetic choice are:

- The patient's medical history
- Level of patient co-operation
- Type of treatment to be provided.

Medical history

In general, local anaesthesia is preferred to general anaesthesia on grounds of safety. For most patients with complicated medical histories, this generalisation is of even greater relevance. Local anaesthesia, unlike general anaesthesia, does not alter the patient's level of consciousness (and impinge on the ability of the patient to maintain their airway). Some factors may, for instance, complicate pre-existing respiratory disease, or require 4–6 hours fasting before treatment (so disrupting blood glucose control in diabetics).

There are few contraindications to local anaesthesia on grounds of medical history. One important example, however, is that of haemophiliacs, when haemorrhage deep in the tissues around the pharynx could follow the injection of an inferior dental block, and thus threaten the patency of the airway. Treatment to replace the deficient clotting factor and/or the use of superficial infiltration injections often overcome the problem without recourse to a general anaesthetic. Occasionally a general anaesthetic is still required.

Further examples of medical conditions which may influence the choice of anaesthetic are given in Table 8.1. When there is any doubt about the suitable choice of anaesthetic, the patient's medical practitioner and/or hospital specialist should be consulted.

Co-operation of the patient

Most patients find most forms of dental treatment under local anaesthesia acceptable. There are, however, some groups of patients with whom the use of local anaesthetic alone does not ensure adequate co-operation so that the dental procedure can proceed safely and effectively. These include:

- Young children below the age of reason
- Mentally handicapped people
- People with dental phobia
- Patients with extreme anxiety.

For the first two groups of patients there may be an indication for general anaesthesia but for the anxious patient, or those with a phobia of dentistry, sedation offers a preferable way of making dental treatment with local anaesthesia an acceptable possibility.

The type of treatment

Local anaesthesia is best suited for operative procedures that are limited both in time, severity, and anatomical extent. Most types of dental treatment fall into this category, but some kinds of dentistry, notably multiple extractions or complex surgical procedures, may test the boundaries of what patients will comfortably tolerate in the fully conscious state. Here again there is an important role for the techniques of intravenous or inhalational sedation to recruit more patients to treatment without a general anaesthetic.

The types of treatment for which local anaesthesia is less well suited:

- Difficult or extensive surgical procedures
- Multiple operative sites in different quadrants of the mouth
- Anatomical sites that are difficult to anaesthetise (e.g. the deep aspect of a dental cyst in the maxilla close to the antrum)
- Drainage of abscesses in deep tissue spaces.

Table 8.1 Medical indications for the use of local anaesthesia

Condition	Clinical problem and tissue system involved	Avoiding action
	CARDIOVASCULAR	
Ischaemic heart disease, e.g. angina, myocardial infarction, coronary artery bypass grafts	Arrhythmias Further ischaemia General anaesthetic risk	Control pain and anxiety Local anaesthetic preferred Consider hospital treatment
Heart failure	Orthopnoea	Sit patient up Local anaesthetic preferred
Thrombo-embolic disease	Deep vein thrombosis Pulmonary embolus	Local anaesthetic preferred Avoid general anaesthetic
	RESPIRATORY	
Asthma	Acute asthmatic attack	Local anaesthetic preferred
Chronic bronchitis Emphysema	General anaesthetic risk – obstructed airways Post-operative chest infection	Use local anaesthetic
Cystic fibrosis Fibrosing alveolitis	General anaesthetic risk – restricted lung volume, poor lung function	Use local anaesthetic
	NERVOUS	
Cerebrovascular accident (stroke)	Further cerebrovascular accident Potential general anaesthetic risk	Use local anaesthetic
Multiple sclerosis	Exacerbation of multiple sclerosis	Use local anaesthetic

GASTRO-INTESTINAL

Condition	Effect	Recommendation
Liver failure	Haemorrhage Impaired drug metabolism	Reduce dosage Local anaesthetic preferred
Inflammatory bowel disease Malabsorption conditions	Steroid therapy (steroid crisis) Anaemia (potential general anaesthetic risk)	Give steroid cover Local anaesthetic preferred

HAEMATOLOGICAL

Condition	Effect	Recommendation
Clotting/platelet disorders (factor VIII) Anticoagulant therapy	Excessive bleeding	Liaise with physician Give factor replacement therapy/reduce anticoagulant therapy Caution with inferior dental block (danger of parapharyngeal haematoma – restriction of airway)
Anaemias, specially sickle cell	General anaesthetic risk	Use local anaesthetic

ENDOCRINE

Condition	Effect	Recommendation
Diabetes mellitus	Hyper- or hypoglycaemia	Use local anaesthetic
Hyperthyroidism	Arrhythmias Thyroid crisis	Avoid adrenaline in local anaesthesia Avoid general anaesthetic
Hypothyroidism	Slow drug metabolism	Local anaesthetic preferred
Pregnancy	Teratogenicity Premature labour	Avoid elective procedures Local anaesthetic preferred (lignocaine and adrenaline)

The choice of anaesthetic technique that is most appropriate for any given patient will depend on a combination of the factors discussed in this chapter. While local anaesthesia is the safest option in the vast majority of cases, there are complications attributable to local anaesthetic agents and the methods of their delivery. These problems are given further consideration in Chapters 9 and 10.

Chapter 9

Local complications

Failure of anaesthesia

The most common reasons for failure of local anaesthesia are:

- Inaccurate placement of the local anaesthetic solution
- Placing too little solution
- Not allowing sufficient time for the solution to diffuse and take effect
- Injection into inflamed tissues
- Using an expired anaesthetic solution.

It is usually better to put in slightly more anaesthetic than necessary, rather than risk failure of the local anaesthetic with the attendant loss of patient confidence. There is a wide safety margin between the effective dose and toxicity, even if it is narrower than formerly believed. In the event of failure, repeating the injection will achieve the necessary anaesthesia. If an anaesthetic has not started to work within 5 minutes it should be repeated. Where a mandibular block has failed to achieve anaesthesia it should be repeated, followed additionally by local infiltration or even intraligamentary anaesthesia in persistent cases. Where maxillary buccal infiltration has not succeeded, a palatal infiltration can be administered as well as repeating the buccal injection (see Chapters 6 and 7.)

Infection

It is recommended that a local anaesthetic should not be placed into infected tissues, because of the risk of spreading the infection. Furthermore, the local anaesthetic is unlikely to be effective, because of the increased local blood flow and a lowering of pH within the infected tissues. Such a situation can normally be managed in the case of a localised abscess, by injecting into the normal tissues around those that are infected, or by using a regional block technique where the injection is at a distant site.

Very occasionally infection may be spread into the tissues by the needle passing through a contaminated tissue surface or by the needle becoming contaminated before use.

Intravascular injection

In the same way in which a blood vessel may be damaged by the tip of a needle causing a haematoma (see later), so may the needle inadvertently be placed in the lumen of a blood vessel. Injection of the solution at this stage results in the contents of the anaesthetic solution (including the vasoconstrictor) passing into the systemic circulation (see Chapter 10). In addition there is failure of the local anaesthetic, as the agent is rapidly removed from the intended site. Aspirating syringes are used to avoid this problem. After placing the needle in position for placement of the anaesthetic, aspirating the syringe will indicate if a vessel has been perforated (Figure 9.1). If so, the needle should be partially withdrawn and re-sited to prevent intravascular injection at this stage.

Haematoma

Occasionally, bleeding into the tissues may follow administration of a local anaesthetic. In normal circumstances following minimal leakage of blood into the extravascular tissues the patient is unaware of the problem. Where there has been significant bleeding into the tissues, a pool of blood will collect, produce a swelling and act as an irritant to the tissues, causing pain and trismus. In theory the localised collection of blood could become an ideal culture medium for bacteria, although infection of such a haematoma is extremely rare. Antibiotics have been recommended, but there is no indication for this unless signs of infection of the haematoma are identified. Given time, the clot will organize and the swelling gradually disappear. In some instances of haematoma formation in the medial pterygoid muscle, active manipulation of the jaw is required to treat the severe trismus that can result.

Nerve damage

Rarely, when giving an injection, particularly a mandibular block, the needle pierces a nerve bundle during placement; this gives an immediate 'electric shock' sensation to the patient. It is usually

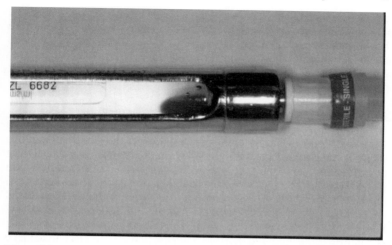

Figure 9.1.   A photograph of the cartridge containing blood aspirated following perforation of a vessel. If this occurs the needle is partially withdrawn and again aspirated. If no new blood is seen the solution is deposited.

followed by partially effective anaesthesia and subsequently a complete return to normal sensation. Rarely are there long-term complications of nerve damage from this event (see Chapter 11).

Needle fracture

Before the use of disposable needles, needle fracture was a recognized complication of re-usable needles, but it is now extremely rare with high quality disposable needles. It is still advisable never to insert a needle into the tissues right up to its hub, as that is where it is weakest. Should a needle break at this point, then the protruding part can be grabbed with artery forceps. If a needle is found to be bent when it is removed from an injection site, it should not be used for another injection on the same patient, but replaced by a fresh needle.

Cartridge failure

Cartridges of local anaesthetic have traditionally been made of glass, and therefore may be damaged in transit or may break if dropped. To overcome this some are now made of polypropylene. Before use, glass cartridges should be examined for damage and discarded if cracked. Cartridges should also be examined to ensure no solution has leaked in transit (a large air bubble being visible). Leakage from the plastic based cartridges during injection is not uncommon and appears to be due mainly to distortion of the bung by inaccurate placement of the plunger.

Facial palsy

If an injection is given in close proximity to the facial nerve then this motor nerve will become paralysed. This may occur when the needle for a mandibular block is placed too far back and enters the capsule of the parotid gland. Various branches of the facial nerve will be affected, with dramatic effect, causing the temporary paralysis of muscles of facial expression (similar to that in Bell's palsy). The effect lasts about 1–2 hours. In these circumstances the trigeminal nerve is not anaesthetised, and a further injection will need to be given in the right place to achieve the desired effect.

Needle-stick injury

If dentists or nurses are careless they may accidentally prick themselves with an unsheathed needle, and risk cross-infection from the patient. The situation is best avoided by never leaving an unsheathed needle on the instrument tray and by routine use of a sheath guard. Should such an accident occur, the wound should be squeezed to encourage bleeding to remove any contaminated fluid, and then it should be washed. Most hospitals, clinics and large practices have a protocol for handling needle-stick injuries: these should be followed. Infection arising from a needle-stick injury is rare, but hepatitis has been reported. All clinical staff should be vaccinated against hepatitis B.

The essential protocol for a practitioner is often dictated by local recommendations but may include:

- Allow the wound to bleed freely
- Assess the hepatitis status of the operator (for the possible use of passive immunisation)
- Assess the hepatitis status of the patient
- Record the incident in both the patient records and a surgery 'Incident Book'.

Chapter 10

Systemic complications

Introduction

Modern local anaesthetics have an enviable safety record, far better than many other commonly used medicines such as aspirin and penicillin. Approximately 70 million local anaesthetics are given annually in the United Kingdom, and yet there have only ever been a handful of deaths reported where the local anaesthetic has been the principal cause or a significant contributing factor. Reactions to injections of local anaesthetics are not uncommon but most of these are minor and reversible. These adverse reactions may be considered under the following headings:

- Reactions related to the injection procedure alone
- Dose-related toxicity of the local anaesthetic
- Dose-independent hypersensitive reactions to the local anaesthetic
- Problems relating to the vasoconstrictor component
- Reactions to other constituents of the local anaesthetic solution.

Reactions related to the injection

Fainting

The most common adverse reaction to injection of a local anaesthetic is the psychomotor reaction of fainting. Most patients about to receive the sharp end of a needle will feel some anxiety and display a degree of autonomic response. This may take the form of a rise in pulse rate and blood pressure due to sympathetic activation, or the lowering of these cardiovascular parameters due to vasovagal syncope resulting in a reduction of cardiac output. Laying the patient flat and elevating the legs is normally sufficient to restore the venous return to the heart, and thereby the blood pressure. Once conscious, the patient may be offered a glucose drink, as many are too nervous to eat anything before they attend for their dental appointment, and thus may be hypoglycaemic. Fainting episodes can be avoided by sympathetic management of the patient, reclining the patient to a supine or semi-recumbent position before the start of treatment and skilful administration of the injection.

Cross-infection

The administration of a local anaesthetic is probably the most invasive aspect of commonly performed restorative dental procedures. Cross-infection with a contaminated needle is therefore a serious risk, but one which should be completely eliminated with the use of disposable sterile needles which are never used for more than one patient. Once the needle has been removed from its protective sheath, care should be taken to avoid the needle contacting anything other than the patient's mucosa at the site of the injection. This is a particular concern where an unguarded needle on a syringe is placed on an instrument tray in contact with some items that, although clean, may not be sterile. Operators should also be aware of the danger of needle-stick injuries to themselves or their assistants. Routine use of a sheath guard minimises this risk.

Infections that could be transmitted from patient to patient:

1. Herpes simplex
2. Hepatitis B and C (other variants have also been identified)
3. Human immunodeficiency virus
4. Creutzfeldt-Jakob disease.

The following precautions for both staff and patients are mandatory:

1. Disposable needles and cartridges to be used on only one patient
2. Autoclave all other instruments
3. Handle instruments carefully (e.g. use of needle guards)
4. Dispose of used needles into containers, which can be sealed and destroyed.

Spreading infection (cellulitis)

Infection within the perioral tissues could be spread into the tissue planes of the head and neck by the passage of a needle through an infected area. To avoid this complication the injection should either be sited away from the infected area using a regional block technique, or the proposed treatment deferred until the infection has been controlled with antibiotic therapy.

Bleeding disorders

Passage of the needle through the tissues may disrupt small blood vessels, potentially causing bleeding and haematoma formation.

Patients who present with a history of bleeding disorders, particularly clotting defects such as haemophilia (Factor VIII), or who have a history of anticoagulant medication, are at risk of developing extensive bruising or a haematoma large enough to distort the tissues. If such a swelling were to develop around the oropharynx in these patients following an inferior dental block, then the airway could be compromised. To prevent this problem, treatment must be coordinated with the patient's haematologist by replacing the missing coagulation factor, after which the patient can be treated as normal.

Endocarditis risk

Most injections into the perioral tissues cause a small and insignificant bacteraemia which is of a much lower magnitude than that resulting from patients biting their teeth together firmly. However, it has been shown that intraligamentary injections can force significant numbers of bacteria into the circulation and therefore this route of administration is contraindicated in patients at risk of infective endocarditis. In patients susceptible to the consequences of a bacteraemia, there is an indication for disinfection of the mucosa prior to injection. Where antibiotic cover is to be given (for instance in the case of tooth extraction), then any bacteraemia resulting from an intraligamentary injection would also be covered, but the use of an antibiotic cover solely for local anaesthesia is not justified.

Route of injection

The placement of local anaesthetic into the tissues via an intra-osseous or an intraligamentary route results in higher plasma concentrations of the local anaesthetic than when an equivalent volume is injected at other perioral sites. This effect, which is due to the direct introduction of the drug into vascular bony spaces, must be considered when calculating the maximum safe dose to avoid toxicity (see below).

However, these injections require a much lower volume of local anaesthetic (approximately 0.2 ml).

Problems related to the local anaesthetic

Local anaesthetics, such as lignocaine, are membrane stabilisers and therefore block nerve conduction (see Chapter 2). This same action is responsible for the adverse toxic effects seen mostly in the central nervous system (CNS) and the heart. In general, CNS toxicity is clinically identified before cardiac symptoms. At low plasma levels local anaesthetics produce an excitatory response with feelings of dizziness, visual and auditory disturbances, apprehension, disorientation and circumoral anaesthesia. As plasma levels rise, some of the features of CNS depression may follow, including drowsiness, slurred speech, convulsions, hypotension, loss of consciousness and respiratory arrest. There may also be circulatory collapse as the result of ventricular fibrillation. In therapeutic doses (plasma levels of 1–3 μg/ml) lignocaine has an anti-arrhythmic effect on the myocardium and is commonly used in the prophylaxis and treatment of acute arrhythmias following myocardial infarction. There is a consensus view that toxic effects begin at a threshold of about 5 μg/ml but there is no linear relationship between the dose given and the blood level achieved. It is stated that the maximum dose for lignocaine in an adult patient is 4.4 mg/kg, equivalent to approximately 300 mg in a patient weighing 70 kg. Each 2.2 ml cartridge of 2% lignocaine contains 40 mg of drug. These maximum dose limits were originally calculated following injection of local anaesthetics into subcutaneous sites around the body, notably the intercostal area and the perineum. From these data it was also deduced that the addition of a vasoconstrictor, such as adrenaline, further increased the volume of local anaesthetic that could safely be injected without reaching toxic plasma levels. However, further study of the uptake of local anaesthetics from perioral injection sites has shown that plasma levels increase more quickly and achieve higher maximum concentrations when the drug is injected submucosally in the mouth, than when it is given subcutaneously elsewhere in the body. Also, the addition of a vasoconstrictor has little effect in limiting the rate and could be therapeutic for cardiac conditions. Therefore the maximum doses originally given for local anaesthetics and which still appear in some drug data sheets have recently been reduced to those shown in Table 10.1.

Table 10.1   Maximum currently recommended doses for a healthy 70 kg person

Local anaesthetic	Maximum dose (mg/kg)	Maximum total dose in adults (mg)	Maximum number cartridges (2.2 ml)
Lignocaine 2%	4.4	300	7 cartridges
Prilocaine 3%	6	400	6 cartridges
Prilocaine 4%	6	400	4.5 cartridges

Cardiovascular disease

Patients with ischaemic heart disease (angina pectoris, myocardial infarction) or previous cardiac surgery, as well as patients with circulatory dysfunction such as cardiac failure, show higher plasma levels of lignocaine when compared with healthy subjects given the same dose. Therefore it is recommended that the maximum safe dose be halved in such patients. Low plasma potassium levels and acidosis also potentiate adverse effects of local anaesthetics on the myocardium.

Liver disease

Patients with reduced hepatic function exhibit abnormal metabolism of amide local anaesthetics, and toxic plasma levels may result because of an inability to metabolise and clear the drug. Dosage levels should be reduced following advice from the patient's physician.

Pseudo-cholinesterase deficiency

Local anaesthetics of the ester type (e.g. procaine) should be avoided in patients who have this rare familial enzyme defect as metabolism of these drugs is impaired. Ester-type local anaesthetics are no longer in routine use for dental procedures.

Methaemoglobinaemia

This rare complication can be caused by a metabolic product of prilocaine that oxidises the ferrous (Fe^{2+}) component of the haem in red blood cells to the ferric state (Fe^{3+}), reducing their oxygen delivering capacity and resulting in tissue hypoxia.

Pregnancy

All local anaesthetics cross the placenta to some degree. Highest concentrations in the foetal circulation follow injection of prilocaine and the lowest follow bupivacaine, with lignocaine inbetween. Bupivacaine, however, is the most cardiotoxic of local anaesthetics and is contra-indicated in pregnancy. Felypressin, which is a derivative of vasopressin and related to oxytocin, has the potential to cause uterine contractions, although this would be extremely unlikely at the low concentration in local anaesthetic; however, it is best avoided during pregnancy. The local anaesthetic of choice during pregnancy is lignocaine with adrenaline.

Drug interactions

- Muscle relaxants may be potentiated by local anaesthetics; this effect has been observed in patients receiving a combination of lignocaine and suxamethonium
- Anticonvulsants, e.g. phenytoin, and other membrane stabilising drugs are potentiated by local anaesthetics. In theory this effect could produce cardiac toxicity although no cases have been reported
- Beta-blockers compete for the same liver enzymes as those which metabolise amide local anaesthetics. Beta-blockers may also reduce hepatic blood flow, and the combination of these effects could lead to an increased plasma level of local anaesthetic
- Metabolism of sulphonamides shares a pathway with prilocaine, and this interaction could affect the potency of either drug. A case of methaemoglobinaemia in a child has been reported where an interaction between a sulphonamide and EMLA cream (a mixture of prilocaine and lignocaine) was considered to be the cause.

Management of serious toxic adverse reaction to local anaesthetic

- Stop the dental treatment
- Call for appropriate medical assistance
- Monitor the patient's vital signs, particularly the respiratory rate, which may be reduced and which is a more sensitive indicator of toxicity than either pulse rate or blood pressure. Pulse oximetry would be helpful
- Administer oxygen if the patient's saturation, monitored by pulse oximeter, is below optimal level
- Be prepared to administer cardiopulmonary resuscitation.

Allergic reactions to local anaesthetics

Allergy to modern amide-type local anaesthetic solutions is exceedingly rare. Allergic reactions to the ester-type local anaesthetics were more frequently encountered when these were routinely used before the introduction of amide-type anaesthetics. Unfortunately it is still the case that many patients are labelled 'allergic' to a local anaesthetic when the reaction suffered is not one of hypersensitivity but is psychomotor; the result of toxicity or of a local iatrogenic effect. In one study [1] where 25 patients, each of whom had suffered a serious adverse reaction following a local anaesthetic, were suspected of being allergic to the local anaesthetic agent, only one patient had a true allergy. In another similar report of 197 cases [2], only three were found to be the result of true hypersensitivity, one of these being a type IV delayed hypersensitivity reaction; two had an immediate type I reaction, one against lignocaine, the other articaine. In each of these patients no associated IgE antibody could be found despite using sensitive radioimmunoassay techniques. The over-riding concern in these patients is that a further challenge with the suspected antigen may precipitate a severe type I hypersensitivity reaction. Therefore each patient with a significant history of either a localised reaction consisting of swelling, erythema, an itchy rash, or systemic features such as dyspnoea, wheezing, widespread skin rash or circulatory collapse should be referred for full immunological investigation. A list of suitable hospital units where this service is available can be obtained from the British Society for Allergy and Clinical Immunology (BSACI) [3], the address of which appears at the end of this chapter.

Briefly, the testing procedure involves immunologically challenging the patient with the suspected antigen, initially via an intradermal route starting with a very dilute solution and working up in concentration. If this excites no reaction then a test subcutaneous dose of the local anaesthetic is administered. By testing different local anaesthetics in this way it is usually possible to find one to which the patient does not react, in the unlikely event that a true allergy is found.

Problems associated with the vasoconstrictor component

There has been, and still remains, some controversy about the use of adrenaline as a vasoconstrictor in local anaesthetic solutions. The safety record of lignocaine 2% plus 1:80,000 adrenaline is exemplary. Perhaps the most commonly encountered adverse effect with the use of adrenaline is its inadvertent injection into a blood vessel. This produces an increase in cardiac output by increasing stroke volume (positive ionotropic response) and heart rate (positive chronotropic response: tachycardia). There is also a vasoconstrictor effect on the peripheral circulation but a compensatory dilatory effect in skeletal muscle. The overall effect on mean blood pressure is for it to fall slightly. Between 10 and 20% of local anaesthetic injections have shown blood in the syringe on aspiration and therefore have the potential to place some of the local anaesthetic intravascularly. However, only a small proportion of these patients show the symptoms of intravascular adrenaline injection, which are palpitations and a feeling of light headedness. The use of aspirating syringes assists the operator in identifying that a blood vessel has been entered before large quantities are injected into the circulation, and so this risk can be minimized.

Adrenaline is a naturally occurring hormone secreted from the adrenal medulla. In normal subjects performing light physical work, plasma concentrations of adrenaline have been measured at around 4 μg/ml, the same concentration as that achieved by a continuous intravenous infusion of adrenaline at the rate of 10 μg/min. Each 2.2 ml cartridge of lignocaine plus 1:80,000 adrenaline contains 25 μg of adrenaline. It is unlikely that the whole of an anaesthetic cartridge would be injected intravascularly, and moreover if the solution is injected slowly then a plasma concentration of 4 μg/ml is unlikely to be exceeded. Anxiety is a potent stimulus for adrenaline secretion and poor local anaesthesia is a potent source of anxiety. It is a clinical impression widely held and supported by research that lignocaine with adrenaline is the most efficacious local anaesthetic, and its effects are superior to solutions without adrenaline. Two separate studies [4,5] have shown a greater rise in pulse rate and blood pressure in patients who were to have teeth extracted when lignocaine without adrenaline was used compared to lignocaine with adrenaline.

There are, however, some conditions in which injecting adrenaline is contraindicated:

- Crescendo angina
- Recent myocardial infarction or coronary artery bypass graft up to 3 months after operation
- Unstable cardiac arrhythmias
- Hyperthyroid states: there is a theoretical risk of potentiation of adrenaline by excessive levels of thyroid hormone (NB: this is not the case in patients taking thyroxine as replacement therapy)
- Patients with phaeochromocytoma (a rare adrenaline secreting tumour of the adrenal gland)

In these patients any rise of plasma adrenaline is undesirable and a local anaesthetic without adrenaline should be chosen.

In patients who are hypertensive, there is no absolute contra-indication to the use of adrenaline. However, some hypertensive patients will be taking medication which could interact with adrenaline (see below). The severe reactions and hypertensive crises that were recorded following local anaesthetic administration in the past were due to the vasoconstrictor noradrenaline, which has a powerful pressor effect on the alpha receptors in the peripheral vasculature. However, unlike adrenaline, it has very little compensatory beta effect on skeletal muscle vessels, and therefore there may be a substantial rise in blood pressure following the use of noradrenaline. Noradrenaline has now been discontinued as a vasoconstrictor in local anaesthetics.

Drug interactions and potential interactions with adrenaline

- Beta-blocking drugs reduce the beta effects of any injected adrenaline and so will accentuate the alpha effects of vasoconstriction, an increase in peripheral resistance leading to a potential rise in blood pressure. The use of adrenaline is not contraindicated in these patients, but the maximum dose of local anaesthetic containing 1:80,000 adrenaline should be limited to three or four cartridges. Slow injection of the solution is recommended in addition to the use of a self-aspirating syringe.
- Non-potassium sparing diuretics may potentiate one effect of adrenaline, which is to lower plasma potassium level. This combination might threaten cardiotoxicity, particularly in the presence of an acidosis.
- Tricyclic antidepressants, in theory, ought to potentiate the effect of adrenaline by blocking the action of the enzyme *catechol ortho-methyltransferase* (COMT). This controls the rate of re-uptake of adrenaline and other catecholamines into nerve cells. In practice it has never been shown that these patients are at an increased risk, and no serious adverse effect has ever been reported. One study [6] showed that volunteers who were taking tricyclic antidepressants, and who were given an intravenous infusion of adrenaline at the rate of 18 µg/min (equivalent to the adrenaline in 1.5 ml of 1:80,000 solution), showed no serious adverse sequelae even after 25 minutes of adrenaline infusion at that rate.
- Monoamine oxidase inhibitors do not interact with adrenaline. These drugs act by increasing the intraneuronal stores of monoamine oxidase and they would not potentiate the effect of exogenous adrenaline. However, a drug such as ephedrine, which acts by releasing adrenaline stores, will have its effect enhanced by monoamine oxidase inhibitors.
- Drugs of abuse such as cocaine and cannabis show some sympathomimetic effects which could be potentiated by exogenously administered adrenaline.

Problems of the vasoconstrictor felypressin

- Felypressin is related to the naturally occurring hormone oxytocin, which causes uterine contraction and initiates labour. Although this effect is weak at the concentrations of felypressin used in local anaesthetic solutions, the drug is best avoided in pregnancy.
- Felypressin has been shown to cause coronary artery vasoconstriction and cardiac arrhythmias, and is thus not a benign alternative to

adrenaline containing local anaesthetic solution in patients with cardiac disease.

Problems of other constituents of the local anaesthetic

Traditionally local anaesthetics used to contain methylparaben as a preservative. This chemical is structurally related to the ester-type local anaesthetics and could act as a hapten to cause allergy. Most modern local anaesthetics are preservative-free and therefore this problem has largely been eradicated. Solutions containing adrenaline require an anti-oxidant such as sodium metabisulphite to preserve the stability of the solution, and a few cases of reaction to this component have been reported.

References

1. Wildsmith, J. A., McKinnon, R. P. and Rae, S. M. (1998). Allergy to local anaesthetic drugs is rare but does occur. *British Dental Journal*, **184**, 507–510.
2. Gall, H., Kaufmann, R. and Kalverman, C. M. (1996). Adverse reactions to local anaesthetics: analysis of 197 cases. *Journal of Allergy and Clinical Immunology*, **97**, 933–937.
3. BSACI Secretariat, 66 Weston Park, Thames Ditton, Surrey, KT7 0HL.
4. Dick, S. P. (1953). Clinical toxicity of epinephrine anaesthesia. *Oral Surgery, Oral Medicine, Oral Pathology*, **6**, 274–278.
5. Vernale, C. A. (1960). Cardiovascular responses to local dental anaesthesia with epinephrine in normotensive and hypertensive subjects. *Oral Surgery, Oral Medicine, Oral Pathology*, **13**, 942–952.
6. Boakes, A. J., Laurence, D. R., Teoh, P. C. *et al.* (1973). Interactions between sympathomimetic amines and antidepressant agents in man. *British Medical Journal*, **849**, 311–315.

Further reading

Cannell, H. (1996). Evidence for safety margins of lignocaine local anaesthetics for peri-oral use. *British Dental Journal*, **181**, 243–249.
Cawson, R. A., Wilson, I. and Whittington, D. R. (1983). The hazards of dental local anaesthetics. *British Dental Journal*, **154**, 253–258.

Chapter 11

Medico-legal considerations

Introduction

It is incumbent upon every dental practitioner to treat his or her patients in an appropriate way, considering both the present needs of the patient and any special precautions demanded by the past medical history. To avoid the criticism of negligence, a competent practitioner must administer such appropriate treatment. The dentist is required to deliver a standard of care equal to that which could reasonably be expected from a group of his or her colleagues. Furthermore the patient should receive adequate information about the proposed treatment so that informed consent for that treatment can be obtained.

Medico-legal complaints arising from the administration of local anaesthetics to patients are few in number, particularly when compared with the recent upward trend in allegations of malpractice concerning restorative dental procedures and oral surgery. There are, however, some particular complications arising directly from the local anaesthetic drugs or their delivery which merit consideration.

Consent

It is normally assumed that patients submit themselves willingly to a local anaesthetic as part of the proposed dental treatment. Most patients' expectations are that they will receive a local anaesthetic to cover any procedure which is likely to produce discomfort or pain; the giving of an anaesthetic injection is taken as routine by most dentists and patients in most circumstances. However, there are some patients who have particular views on the style of anaesthesia they should receive and even the type of drug that should be used. This may be especially so where patients have suffered some previous adverse reaction, which they associate with a particular compound in the local anaesthetic solution. Although the vast majority of these adverse reactions are not an allergic response, the patient's perception may be that as they have reacted badly they are in some way 'allergic' to it (Chapter 10).

Therefore taking a careful history in these cases and where necessary obtaining old dental records can be extremely helpful in elucidating the facts surrounding previous adverse events, and may help to avoid any recurrence. This procedure may include referring the patient for further investigation of the allergy. There are other ways of avoiding potential problems, e.g. in the choice of local anaesthetic.

With regard to the broader issue of consent, to explain the nature of the treatment about to be given is both sound medico-legal practice and good for rapport with the patient. The treatment includes giving the patient a local anaesthetic injection. Consent to a procedure must be accompanied by an understanding of the procedure; understanding the procedure goes a long way towards allaying fear.

Nerve damage

Persisting anaesthesia or paraesthesia involving branches of the trigeminal nerve is a not uncommon complication following various dental surgical procedures, notably lower third molar removal. There is, however, a small group of patients who may have some sensory loss of the lingual nerve, or less commonly the inferior alveolar nerve following inferior dental block injections for restorative procedures where no surgery is carried out. These cases occasionally present as a legal complaint.

In a survey of over 12,000 inferior dental block injections [1], all given for restorative treatment, 18 patients (0.15%) were found to have some lingual sensory disturbance following their treatment. Of these, 17 patients regained total normal sensation within 6 months and one patient (0.008%) still had a loss of sensation after 1 year. Of the 12,000 patients, 856 (7%) experienced an 'electric shock' type feeling in the tongue at the time of the injection, suggesting that the tip of the anaesthetic needle had touched the lingual nerve. Interestingly, in this series none of the 18 patients with persisting sensory deficit experienced an 'electric shock' at the time of injection. In a further report [2] of almost 10,000 inferior dental block injections, some form of traumatic episode (electric shock type feeling) during the injection was noted in 206 patients (3.6%). Of these 41 went on to report some post-injection sensory deficiency in the tongue. In this study all patients with a persisting numbness or paraesthesia had had an 'electric shock' incident at the time of the injection. In a third study [3] 143 cases of persisting sensory deficit following inferior dental block injections were reported. Out of these 143 patients, 31 had experienced an 'electric shock' at the time of the injection. A further factor in the aetiology of this post-anaesthetic nerve damage was identified in this report. It was noted that the number of cases of post-anaesthetic sensory loss reported with the use of prilocaine or articaine was much higher than that expected from the relative incidence of the use of these anaesthetics. It was pointed out that local neurotoxicity may be one aetiological factor and the authors further commented that these two local anaesthetic substances are the only ones which are presented as a 4% solution. All other local anaesthetic solutions are less concentrated. Among these reports the overall incidence of any persisting nerve damage varied widely, the highest being 1 in 700 injections and the lowest 1 in almost 800,000 injections.

Spectrum of medico-legal complaints arising from local anaesthesia

In a recent survey carried out by one of the authors, records of the Medical Defence Union were examined over a 3-year period and the following complications related to the use of local anaesthetics were noted. This collection of problems represents only those events that formed the basis of complaints by patients and is therefore not exhaustive.

Ineffective local anaesthetic

Six patients complained that the local anaesthetic had worked inadequately to the point where their treatment was distressingly painful.

Fainting (vaso-vagal attack)

Four patients had fainted in the dental chair following the administration of a local anaesthetic, and two of these people had still felt faint as they left the surgery at the end of their appointment.

Painful administration of local anaesthetic

Three patients complained of pain at the time of the injection or undue pain shortly afterwards.

Consent

Three patients stated that they had not given their consent to a local anaesthetic injection.

Broken needle

In two cases local anaesthetic needles, which were subsequently shown to be defective, had fractured at the hub, leaving the fractured portion of the needle in the tissues.

Cardiac arrest

Two patients suffered a cardiac arrest during their dental treatment, both having received local anaesthetic injections of prilocaine. Both patients had ischaemic heart disease previously noted in their medical history and one patient was almost 90 years old.

Local anaesthetic not given

One patient was concerned that a local anaesthetic had not been given at a dental visit which included a root canal treatment, during which the patient experienced some pain.

'Electric shock' in tongue

One patient reported feeling a sharp twinge like an 'electric shock' in the tongue, suggesting that the tip of the needle had touched the lingual nerve during administration of an inferior dental block. This patient did not report any persisting problem.

Swelling and bruising

One patient developed a swollen face within hours of the injection and subsequently was noted to have formed a haematoma at the injection site with bruising on the skin of the cheek.

Wrong solution injected

In one case a patient had been given an injection of non-sterile water which had been placed in a cartridge similar to those used for local anaesthetics.

Wrong injection site

One patient had received a left inferior dental block when a right dental block should have been given.

It is notable that so few medico-legal complaints have arisen out of the vast number of patients who would have received local anaesthetics from members of a defence organisation during this 3-year period. These instances do not of course represent an accurate record of adverse effects, merely the number that were reported as potential medico-legal claims. Sixteen of the 25 cases were related to the following: local anaesthetic had been ineffective, the patient had fainted following its administration, the injection itself was painful, or the patient had failed to give consent to local anaesthesia. These problems should all be avoidable, and have been considered in the preceding chapters. Indeed the same is true of most of the other complaints such as injections given at the wrong site or injecting the wrong solution; actions which are plainly indefensible.

The problem of disturbing the lingual nerve with the tip of the injection needle can be seen as a result of accurate placement of the needle during the administration of an inferior dental block. It is not possible to avoid this complication intentionally and indeed it could be said that the lingual and inferior dental nerves are the target of the injection and therefore a 'direct hit' implies sound knowledge of anatomy. Fortunately the vast majority of these cases resolve spontaneously with no permanent loss of sensation in the areas supplied by the nerves involved.

In both cases where the injection needle fractured, the needle itself was found to be defective with a weakness at the point where it was inserted into the hub. In one case the needle had been inserted into the tissues right up to the hub, and so there was no chance of retrieving the retained portion after it fractured. Although modern local anaesthetic needles are extremely durable and most unlikely to fracture, it is prudent practice not to insert the needle fully into the tissues.

In the two cases where the patients suffered cardiac arrest and died, they were both elderly with known ischaemic heart disease documented in their medical history, and neither patient was given an excessive dose of local anaesthetic. Indeed both patients received prilocaine with felypressin and the total dose was less than three cartridges, well within accepted safety limits.

References

1. Krafft, T. C., and Hickel, R. (1994). Clinical investigation into the incidence of direct damage to the lingual nerve caused by local anaesthesia. *Journal of Craniomaxillofacial Surgery,* **22,** 294–296.
2. Harn, S. D., and Durham, T. M. (1990). Incidence of lingual nerve trauma and post-injection complications in conventional mandibular block anaesthesia. *Journal of the American Dental Association,* **121,** 519–523.
3. Haas, D. A., and Lennon, D. (1995). A 21-year retrospective study of reports of paraesthesia following local anaesthetic administration. *Journal of the Canadian Dental Association,* **61,** 319–350.

Glossary of terms

Anterior superior alveolar nerve. A terminal branch of the maxillary division of the trigeminal nerve supplying the tissues of the premaxilla.

Aspiration. The retraction of the plunger in the barrel of a syringe to establish if a blood vessel has been entered by the needle.

Dental Panoramic Tomograph (DPT). A rotational tomogramic radiograph, used for a general survey of the dentition. This view also demonstrates specific aspects of local anatomy.

Incisive nerve. A terminal branch of the mandibular division of the trigeminal nerve, within the mandibular body, supplying the incisor teeth, given off after the mental nerve leaves via the mental foramen.

Inferior dental nerve (inferior alveolar nerve). One of the largest branches of the mandibular division of the trigeminal nerve, responsible for the majority of sensory innervation of the mandible. It enters the mandible via the mandibular foramen.

Infiltration anaesthesia. The blockade of the terminal branches of a sensory nerve usually in close proximity to the tissues to be anaesthetised.

Infra-orbital nerve. A terminal branch of the maxillary division of the trigeminal nerve which leaves the maxilla by the infra-orbital foramen. This is situated just below the rim of the orbit.

Lingual nerve. A sensory branch of the mandibular nerve. It carries sensory information from the lingual tissues (including the sensation of taste).

Long buccal nerve. A terminal branch of the mandibular division of the trigeminal nerve, responsible for carrying sensory information from the tissues buccal to the mandibular molar teeth.

Mental nerve. A terminal branch of the interior dental nerve of the trigeminal nerve, which leaves the mandible by the foramen found close to the apices of the mandibular premolar teeth, the mental foramen.

Middle superior alveolar nerve. A terminal branch of the maxillary division of the trigeminal nerve supplying the tissues in the mid palalatal region of the alveolar; usually the second premolar and the serial root of the first molar.

Motor nerves. Nerve fibres connecting with skeletal/striated muscle via neuromuscular junctions (motor end plates), which are responsible for initiating a contraction within the muscle fibre. Information passes from the central nervous system to the periphery via these fibres.

Myelin sheath. This insulates the nerve and prevents current flow. The underlying nerve is, however, exposed at certain sites known as 'nodes of Ranvier'.

Pain. An unpleasant sensory and emotional experience associated with actual or potential tissue damage and often described in terms of such damage. Certain 'defensive' behaviours are associated with pain to prevent/reduce tissue damage.

Posterior superior alveolar nerve. A terminal branch of the maxillary division of the trigeminal nerve supplying the tissues of the posterior maxilla.

Pterygomandibular raphe. A decussation of muscle fibres found medial to the site of injection for an inferior dental regional nerve block. It consists of fibres from the buccinator muscle on the lateral aspect and the superior constrictor of the pharynx on the medial aspect.

Regional block anaesthesia. The placement of local anaesthetic solution proximal to the site required and blockading many peripheral nerve fibres. A larger area of tissue is blocked by one injection than is the case with infiltration anaesthesia.

Saltatory conduction. This is the mechanism by which nerves appear to conduct changes in potential whereby the voltage jumps from one node of Ranvier to the next, and in so doing increases the speed of conduction. Depolarisation of the nerve effectively jumps from node to node and is called saltatory conduction. It serves to increase the speed of conduction by approximately 50 times that of unmyelinated fibres.

Sensory nerves. Those nerve fibres which carry the five senses (smell, sight, touch, hearing and taste) and specific subconscious information from the periphery of the body to the central nervous system. Within the broad description of touch are other subcategories: temperature, pressure and, at specific levels, pain.

Synapse. The mechanism which passes information from one nerve fibre to another, being either excitatory or inhibitory. A unique property of synapses is that they only allow a unidirectional flow of information.

Index

Page numbers printed in **bold** type refer to figures; those in *italic* to tables. Page numbers preceded by an asterisk (*) refer to glossary entries.